TU
BAC
TIME

DR AAMER KHAN
WITH CAROLE MALONE

TURN BACK TIME

LOSE WEIGHT AND KNOCK YEARS OFF YOUR AGE

JB
JOHN BLAKE

Published by John Blake Publishing Ltd,
3 Bramber Court, 2 Bramber Road,
London W14 9PB, England

www.johnblakebooks.com

www.facebook.com/johnblakebooks
twitter.com/jblakebooks

This edition published in 2017

ISBN: 978 1 78606 827 9

British Library Cataloguing-in-Publication Data:

A catalogue record for this book is available from the British Library.

Design by www.envydesign.co.uk

Printed in Great Britain by Clays Ltd, St Ives plc

1 3 5 7 9 10 8 6 4 2

Papers used by John Blake Publishing are natural, recyclable products made from wood grown in sustainable forests. The manufacturing processes conform to the environmental regulations of the country of origin.

John Blake Publishing is an imprint of Bonnier Publishing
www.bonnierpublishing.com

CONTENTS

The information provided in this book is designed to provide helpful information on the subjects discussed and is based on the breadth and wealth of Dr Aamer Khan's medical experience since becoming a qualified doctor over thirty years ago.

This book is not meant to be used, nor should it be used, to diagnose or treat any medical condition. For diagnosis or treatment of any medical problem, consult your own physician. The publisher and authors are not responsible for any specific health or allergy needs that may require medical supervision and are not liable for any damages or negative consequences from any treatment, action, application or preparation, to any person reading or following the information in this book. References are provided for informational purposes only and do not constitute endorsement of any websites or other sources.

Readers should be aware that the websites listed in this book may change.

PREFACE

WHY I WROTE THIS BOOK BY DR AAMER KHAN

Hello, my name is Dr Aamer Khan. I am a medical doctor. In 1986 I qualified from The Medical School of the University of Birmingham. I knew that I wanted to be a doctor since the age of eight years old, being inspired by the stories my father told me about my grandfather, who was a surgeon. I have always wanted to help people improve their health and daily lives and have dedicated myself to medicine since taking, and sticking to, the Hippocratic Oath on qualifying.

There are nine undertakings in the Hippocratic Oath:

'I swear to fulfil, to the best of my ability and judgement, this covenant:

1. I will respect the hard-won scientific gains of those physicians in whose steps I walk, and gladly share such knowledge as is mine with those who are to follow.
2. I will apply, for the benefit of the sick, all measures [that] are required, avoiding those twin traps of overtreatment and therapeutic nihilism.
3. I will remember that there is art to medicine as well as science, and that warmth, sympathy, and understanding may outweigh the surgeon's knife or the chemist's drug.
4. I will not be ashamed to say 'I know not,' nor will I fail to call in my colleagues when the skills of another are needed for a patient's recovery.
5. I will respect the privacy of my patients, for their problems are not disclosed to me that the world may know. Most especially must I tread with care in matters of life and death. If it is given me to save a life, all thanks. But it may also be within my power to take a life; this awesome responsibility must be faced with great humbleness and awareness of my own frailty. Above all, I must not play at God.
6. I will remember that I do not treat a fever chart, a cancerous growth, but a sick human being, whose illness may affect the person's family and economic stability. My responsibility includes these related problems, if I am to care adequately for the sick.

7. I will prevent disease whenever I can, for prevention is preferable to cure.
8. I will remember that I remain a member of society, with special obligations to all my fellow human beings, those sound of mind and body as well as the infirm.
9. If I do not violate this oath, may I enjoy life and art, respected while I live and remembered with affection thereafter. May I always act so as to preserve the finest traditions of my calling and may I long experience the joy of healing those who seek my help.'

It is with respect to the seventh and eighth obligations of this oath that I have undertaken research and have come to writing this guide for turning back time and recreating a healthy body, mind and psychological health that everybody can use and benefit from.

When my wife Lesley and I decided to enter a new era of our lives, and career in aesthetic and anti-ageing medicine in Harley Street, London, we began to realise that it wasn't enough just to help people look better and younger on the outside. We realised that in order to look and feel good we had to encompass the whole person's internal health and help to improve them both inside and out. We also realised that what we were actually practicing was not just cosmetic medicine and surgery, but internal and anti-ageing medicine. Looking good is not enough if you still have aches and pains associated with ageing and you can't walk properly, or even get in and out of a taxi. Living life with pain always shows on your face.

About eight years ago we decided to study the subject of Ageing and Human Physiology. I was astonished by how much medical research had already been done, but was not common knowledge. I was just as astounded by the desire of people to look and feel good, and to stay younger for longer, and have healthier, more productive and useful lives. This desire is a bigger drive than the desire to simply look better on the outside. What I found was that by slowing down, and even reversing the ageing process, people don't just feel better, they also look younger.

Clinical research has also shown that most of the age-related disease processes are related to the process of ageing itself and if we slow that down, or even reverse it, we can improve these conditions. It used to be thought that 80 per cent of our outcome was genetic and 20 per cent was due to the environment, so medicine has developed to focus on managing disease processes and their symptoms through prescribing medicines and operating on the end results of these medical conditions. In actuality, we have discovered genetics only determine 20 per cent of the outcome and 80 per cent is determined by our environment; this has led to more and more medical focus on preventing, delaying and curing medical conditions at a much earlier stage.

How we look on the outside reflects what is going on inside. When our systems start to fail we develop outward signs of ageing, which include obesity, muscular and joint stiffness and inflammation, aches and pains, ageing and coarseness of skin, dull eyes, thinning and greying of hair, changes in visual acuity and mental changes, with poor concentration, memory loss, feelings of anxiety, depression, dread and poor sleep.

In a desire to improve their health, people have tried various diets, exercise and nutritional programmes without much success, and at great cost to their pockets, which often even accelerate the very processes that they are trying to slow down. Clinical studies of such programmes have shown that none of them work. Most people who I have come across tend to say that these programmes are so extreme that they are not sustainable. They do not allow for a normal lifestyle, where we have to work, live as part of a family and socialise. For some people, the cost may be prohibitive, or they just don't have the time. A lot of the programmes make people feel worse and they just give up on them. I have found that there is a great deal of confusion about how to achieve good health and which programme is best.

So I wanted to produce a book that would serve as a total body service manual, giving people the simple tools and the knowledge required to use them, so they could make a significant, sustainable difference to their health and wellbeing that could reverse their ageing, and possibly extend their lives by fifteen good-quality years, maybe even more.

I had two other light-bulb moments that further inspired and drove me to write this book:

- About fifteen years ago I decided to develop a nutritionally based health plan that looked at diet, nutrition and exercise based on cellular physiology and health. I tested it on hundreds of people and found that it helped them achieve better health, with a better weight control, less inflammation, and better physical and mental functioning. Those with medical conditions such as arthritis, high blood pressure, diabetes and thyroid problems found that their control of these conditions was improved with the medication they were taking. People also reported an improvement in their night vision while driving.

- About ten years ago, when my wife and I decided to start our Harley Street Practice, we used to travel from Birmingham to London and back on the days we were working in Harley Street. I also had a NHS practice in Birmingham, and Lesley had a cosmeceutical company and rooms in Harley Street. We would get up at 5am and leave at 6.30. I would stop for fuel, and by the time I had filled the car, paid for it and got back in, Lesley would be fast asleep. I thought she was just tired because of the hours and energy we were putting into our business.

Lesley then started to gain weight and complain of pains in her feet. As a medical doctor these should have been red flags to me for something not being quite right. Had a patient presented with these symptoms, I would have immediately got into diagnosing what was going wrong with them. Lesley and I were so close that I missed the early signs and it wasn't until she reported hair loss that I thought of investigating her for an underactive thyroid, which she had.

After this I asked myself the question: if I, a qualified doctor with over twenty years' experience, at that time, of diagnosing and treating these conditions could miss the early signs of such a condition in someone who is so close and important to me, then how many people are out there who are living with the early signs of a medical condition related to their lifestyles, and justifying and rationalising the signs and symptoms as those of inevitable ageing?

Sometimes we are so close to the Elephant, all we see is 'Grey'.

I want to be able to help people pick up on and recognise the early signs of things going wrong, and change the course of their health and highlight it to their GPs at an early stage. I would like this book to help people understand the ageing process – what accelerates it, how that is related to disease processes and what can be done to reverse and slow it down – so they can improve their physical, psychological and mental health and wellbeing.

I dedicate this book to my loving wife, who is a constant support and inspiration to me in all that I do, and to our six wonderful children, Luke, Adam, Farooq, Nadia, Sophie, and Sophia who have brought so much joy into our lives.

INTRODUCTION

From the time we are born our bodies are determined by our genetic blueprint and controlled by various hormones and growth factors, which determine our growth, maturation and development. Most people reach their peak functioning by the age of about thirty years. The growth hormones and factors change and start to diminish from our mid-twenties, and from our mid-thirties we start to age. During our younger, vital years our hormones and growth factors offer protection against environmental hazards and our defences and ability to repair are strong. Our gut bacteria are healthy and work with our bodies to develop a strong and stable immune system that protects our health and wellbeing.

After the age of thirty-five years, our master control hormones change and our bodies start to age, and environmental factors start to have more of an influence on the body. The gut bacteria have probably been damaged by thirty-five years of poor diet and antibiotic exposure, either from prescribed antibiotics, or the antibiotics present in the food chain, so our immune system is compromised, damaged, or, worse still, attacking the host. This is one of the reasons why cancers in younger people are more aggressive and grow and spread more quickly. It is also why cancers accelerate during pregnancy as the growth factors and hormones surge.

The change in the hormones and growth factors can be seen partially as a protective change, as high levels of growth hormone and growth factors in later life would further accelerate any cancers or speed up the ageing process in damaged cells. This would include supercharging any abnormal activity by a damaged immune system. In simple terms, our internal environment influences our health, vitality and wellbeing up to the age of thirty-five and our external environment influences them thereafter. This is assuming we lead a healthy lifestyle and do not poison or damage our internal system. There are a number of factors that affect health outcomes:

Genetics

There is a lot of misconception about the importance of genetics versus environment in the ageing process. Overall, genetics accounts for 20 per cent towards ageing, and non-genetic factors 80 per cent. This does not take into consideration specific genetic or congenital conditions that can lead to shortened life expectancy.

We have genetic tests available that can predict risk factors, which we can then address through very specific lifestyle and environmental changes. Genetic studies in certain groups of people with genetic peculiarities have shown that the presence or absence of certain genes are associated with the slowing or stopping of the ageing process. This is associated with the absence of degenerative, or age-related disease processes like dementia, diabetes, heart disease and even cancer.

Diet and nutrition

Diet provides us with nutrition, energy and external growth factors that work with and complement our internal systems that affect our metabolism, repair and vitality. Food also introduces new organisms, genetic material and antibiotics (these are not listed on the list of ingredients on the packaging) that affect our internal gut bacterial balance, metabolism and can even increase the risk of cancer. As we age we need to consider that the foods that were good for us up to the age of thirty-five may actually accelerate the ageing process so we need to change how and what we eat as we get older.

Exercise

We all know that exercise is important. However, the type and intensity of exercise has to be tailored to our age and, to a lesser degree, genetic/metabolic makeup. Intense, heavy and prolonged exercise that is tolerated by a younger body can be detrimental as we get older and can indeed speed up ageing, degeneration, fat retention and accelerate disease processes, including cancer.

Gut bacterial balance

There is overwhelming evidence to show that the gut microbiome has a very important part to play in regulating the immune system and protecting us from diseases. The microbiome communicates with our central nervous system and can affect our mood, causing feelings of depression and cravings.

There are over 1,000 species of micro-organisms

in the gut, consisting of over 3 million genes, which are important to our wellbeing. They perform many functions other than regulating our immune system. These include aiding in digestion and presentation of vitamins and minerals for absorption, regulation of metabolism and the prevention of obesity. Once upset, these regulatory functions can be affected, resulting in autoimmune diseases, metabolic diseases, obesity and gut problems, and even cancer (lymphoma). Other conditions linked to upset gut bacteria include mental and psychological conditions, like anxiety disorder and depression.

It is not just the gut where such useful micro-organisms are found, but also in the mouth, in the vagina and on the skin, where they play a crucial role in the health of that area, and the defence from harmful elements in the external environment. These 'friendly' organisms are so generous that they have donated DNA that forms the mitochondria that act as energy generators for each and every cell in the human body. We now have means of testing for every bacterial gene in the gut from a simple stool test and this will, in the near future, be able to help us to treat and prevent illness, and reverse the ageing process.

Lifestyle, learning and habits

Long-term studies looking at twins and people's habits, lifestyles and even education (including the way they learn), have given insights into how these affect the way we age internally, how our brains regress and how we can reverse these changes. Some of these studies started over seventy years ago. We also have access to blood and DNA tests that can tell us what our physiological, or biological age is, and how we can reverse it.

CHAPTER 1

THE TIPPING POINT

To understand what happens with ageing, we can study what we see in nature. Every year we see the garden develop and grow; it then reaches maturity before dying out towards the end of the year. In the same way humans are born, then grow and develop, they then stop growing and start to grow old and die. Life is a cycle of growth and decay. The 'Tipping Point' is when we stop growing and start to age. For humans this occurs in our mid-thirties.

When we are young and in the growth and development state the master hormones are growth hormone and the sex hormones. These stimulate tissue growth and vitality and help cells to turn over, stimulating our systems to develop. We have an incredible resilience to the environment – we can eat what we want, to a degree, and our bodies just bounce back after any injury. There is a downside to this in that any tumours or diseases that develop in our younger years are also stimulated and accelerated by the effects of growth hormones. This is also seen during pregnancy, when there is a high level of growth hormones circulating. Fortunately, though, these conditions are very rare at a young age.

In our early years our bodies and systems resist the environmental effects so we appear to be able to get away with a less healthy lifestyle. Our bodies also have a requirement for a varied diet of meat, vegetables and fruits and nuts. These dietary elements appear to help us maintain a strong and healthy system during the regenerative and growth stage of our lives.

As we get closer to the 'Tipping Point' our growth hormone levels naturally decline as we enter the ageing phase of our lives. This is nature's way of protecting us as high levels of growth hormones will accelerate the ageing process and we would burn out more quickly. Also, we produce more abnormal cells with age that can lead to cancer, and growth hormone will accelerate the development of cancer and any other disease condition. We also become more responsive to our environment and diet. This means that we need to change what and how we eat, and how we exercise as we get older. After the 'Tipping Point' we are more sensitive to insulin and cortisol, as our dominating hormones, and these have more of a metabolic effect.

Though the 'Tipping Point' for men and women is the same, women experience the symptoms of hormonal imbalances earlier than men do, from their mid-thirties, and men from their mid-forties. Symptoms of hormonal imbalance and system upset include:

- weight gain
- increase in abdominal fat
- loss of muscle and bone mass
- stiffness, aches and pains of the bones, muscles and joints
- low sex drive
- tiredness and sweating
- poor sleep
- irritability, anxiety and feelings of depression
- digestive problems, with heartburn, bloating and cravings
- acceleration of the signs of ageing in the face and body

There is a change in the hormonal balance, and so in the way the body works and interacts with the environment – what worked for us in our twenties will not necessarily work in our forties or fifties.

The above situation has always been so, however, we

now have another problem to contend with, which has made things even harder. It has resulted in the increase in the incidence of obesity, heart disease, high blood pressure, dementia, diabetes, cancer and other diseases related to ageing, and leading to poor health, suffering and premature death. This new problem is the effect of how and what we eat, how we exercise and the changes we have seen in our environment.

Even in our early stages of life our systems are being damaged by our 'toxic' environment, including:

- pollution
- processed foods
- modern farming techniques in agriculture and livestock management
- high levels of stress
- the trends of yo-yo dieting and weight fluctuations
- repeated use of antibiotics, including the antibiotics we ingest in our food and those we are prescribed
- use of recreational drugs
- use of cigarettes and alcohol
- higher stress levels in our lives
- changes in our working environments
- less time for exercise and recreation; less time for people and social interaction

Interestingly, the word 'recreation' comes from the Latin word '*recreare*', meaning 'create again, renew', via the old French Latin word '*recreatio*', to mean 'mental or spiritual consolation' in late Middle English.

By understanding how the body works, and what and how things can go wrong, we can make lifestyle changes to prevent health deterioration and improve matters. Our body is an incredible vehicle that has developed and evolved over centuries to survive in the environment in which we live. We live in a delicate balance with millions of microorganisms that live in our guts, on our skins, in our mouths and in the vaginas of women; that work in harmony to create a healthy immune and healing system, protecting us from nasty (or pathogenic) infections and helping us to recognise and repair any damage or abnormal cells.

The evidence shows that we carry more than 2kg of microorganisms, with over 1,000 species in our guts. Similarly, there are over 1,000 species of microorganism that live on the skin. These account for over 3 million genes. We also know that over two-thirds of the microbes are unique and individual to the person, and they work with the host to modify the immune system and prevent autoimmune and inflammatory conditions. Some of them have been shown to have a role in the production and absorption of certain vitamins that play a part in the immune system.

Research has also identified that the absence of certain microbes is associated with metabolic disease, such as type 2 diabetes and obesity. There is also a link with microbial upset and the development of certain cancers, anxiety and depression, and autism in children. There is also a strong link with microbial upset and immune conditions, such as eczema, thyroid disease, and other autoimmune conditions.

Our toxic environment is harming our tiny friends, which, in turn, is creating problems with our health. It is important to know how to look after our little allies while we are young, so they can look after us as we grow older. A good way to look at these microbes is as 'guards' that protect our bodies against external harmful factors. They also work with our immune system (our internal soldiers) to protect and repair our bodies. We know that over millions of years our bacterial friends have not just worked with us, but have also given up their attributes to allow us to develop as human beings. The very mitochondria that are the power plants for each cell, and without which we would not be able to survive, originate from bacteria, and carry their own DNA composition. By ensuring our existence, they also ensure their own existence, by having a symbiotic existence with us. We are like a supervessel for them to live in and on in symbiotic harmony.

CHAPTER 2

FAT: FRIEND OR FOE?

Fat in our body and in our diet has a number of important roles. I decided to write this chapter because there is a great deal of confusion about fat, and many diets and exercise programmes are designed around this subject, which can be harmful to health and wellness. I hope this chapter will help to demystify the subject.

IMPORTANT ROLES OF FAT IN OUR BODY

Provision of energy

Although carbohydrates form the main source of energy for our bodies, fat is a source of back-up energy, when carbohydrates are not readily available. One gram of fat has nine calories, compared with four calories per gram of carbohydrates and proteins, and seven calories per gram of alcohol.

Helps absorb and store fat-soluble vitamins

Certain vitamins require fat as a carrier to be absorbed into the body. These are known as 'fat-soluble vitamins'. They are also stored in the fat in the body. These include vitamins A, D, E and K, which are essential for a healthy body and immune and circulatory system.

Energy storage

Consumption of food surplus to the body's needs is stored in the form of fat. Fat stores are found under the skin. Fat is also deposited around organs and this can act as energy storage too.

Insulation

Fat acts an insulation under the skin, maintaining the internal temperature. The deeper skin layers then insulate the core against extreme temperature changes. It also has a thermogenic effect: this is where it can generate and release heat when our skin temperature drops significantly.

Protection

Fat is organised to form cushions around major organs, to act like shock absorbers and protective pads.

Detoxification

Body fat helps to eliminate, store and excrete toxins and certain drugs from the rest of the body.

Hormonal function

Fat cells regulate the production of the sex hormones, particularly oestrogen. Fat is also a component of prostaglandins (hormones produced by individual cells), which have a regulatory role in the body, particularly on platelets and clotting; the uterus, in regulating conception, pregnancy and labour; in modulating the immune system and the inflammatory response; controlling fluid transfer in the guts; controlling electrolyte balance in the kidneys; controlling blood pressure and in the metabolism of fat. They also have a role in the transmission of pain, controlling intraocular pressure in glaucoma, regulating the movement of calcium, controlling cell growth, producing fever during an infection, inhibiting acid production and increasing libido.

They can also cause constriction and dilatation of the airways. As you can see, these are one of the most crucial substances found in the body, with hormone-like and regulatory functions on the body's systems.

Cellular health and integrity

Fat is an essential part of the cell membrane (wall), which plays an important role in keeping each cell healthy and functioning correctly.

Brain and nervous system

Fat forms the structural components of the brain and the nervous system. It is the basis of the myelin sheath, which helps transmit the nerve signals quickly.

Maintenance of mood

Fat in our diet releases endorphins, which stimulate the pleasure centres. It also enhances the taste of food that we eat.

THE STORY OF FAT

The distribution of fat in the body is determined by our genetics. The number of fat cells in our bodies is determined by our diets during childhood, and once set, the number and type of fat cells remain the same throughout life. The amount of fat stored in our fat cells is then determined by our surplus calorie intake and hormonal action, particularly after the age of thirty-five.

Below thirty-five our metabolism and health is mainly driven by our genetic blueprint. After the age of thirty-five, which I refer to throughout as the 'Tipping Point', our environment and lifestyle has a greater role on our metabolism, weight and health. This is related to our cellular health.

We know that cells become less efficient with age, which is partly due to hormonal changes, and partly due to our environment, which includes free radical damage, toxic damage, poor nutrition and inefficient fuel usage by the cells, i.e. carbohydrates. There produce toxic end products and free radicals as a by-product of metabolism rather than medium chain fatty acids, which are a much cleaner source of fuel for cells.

THE HORMONES THAT AFFECT FAT METABOLISM

- **Insulin – known as the number 1 fat storer**
  Insulin is strongly influenced by foods that increase blood sugar. Blood sugar is toxic and about 90 per cent is removed from the blood in two minutes, and stored as glycogen or fat by insulin.

A persistently poor diet, with overconsumption of calories such as carbohydrates, fats or protein – which chronically stimulates the release of insulin – will eventually lead to insulin resistance and ultimately results in the development of metabolic syndrome and diabetes. Insulin resistance results in high levels of insulin, which inhibits the fat-burning effects of other hormones.

- **Glucagon – known as the number 1 fat burner**
  Glucagon has the opposite effect to insulin, but is inhibited by chronically high levels of insulin. By controlling insulin levels, we can allow glucagon to do its work and help burn fat.

- **Ghrelin and Leptin – known as the hunger hormones**
  These work to increase and decrease appetite. Both respond to dietary and exercise stress so we can manipulate them and control our weight gain or loss without resorting to potentially harmful slimming drugs and supplements.

- **Ghrelin – the hunger hormone that increases appetite**
  This peptide hormone (considered to be a growth hormone releasing peptide, or GHR) is secreted

by the stomach and sends signals to the brain that causes you to feel hungrier. Its levels rise before and drop after meals. It is therefore a fast-acting hormone.

Ghrelin has metabolic effects, in that it controls insulin and leptin sensitivity (resulting in insulin and leptin resistance); it also stimulates growth hormone and growth peptides. In cases of a dilated stomach the secretion of ghrelin becomes excessive and out of control because the stomach stretch response is lost, which means that it overrides the signals from the gut to the brain that tell you to stop eating (satiatory response). It has been shown to play a role in short-term feeding and long-term weight gain.

Ghrelin can be seen as a 'gremlin' that plays havoc with other hormones and the body's metabolism by influencing:

1. Regulation of growth hormone, insulin and leptin secretion and sensitivity
2. Glucose and lipid metabolism
3. Gut motility
4. Blood pressure and heart rate
5. Slowing of metabolism and thermogenesis (the efficiency of mitochondria to produce energy and heat), so less energy is released by cells.

Stress also stimulates ghrelin production, thereby increasing the tendency to snack and overeat.

- **Leptin – the hunger hormone that reduces appetite, which acts like a fuel gauge**
  This peptide hormone is produced by fat cells and decreases appetite by communicating how much fat is stored and available to burn to the brain. It also has a long-term regulatory role with energy balance management, inducing weight loss. Leptin influences thyroid hormonal activity to manage metabolism.

  It works on the same part of the brain as ghrelin, but has opposite effects. People who have higher fat levels produce more leptin, however they tend to have a leptin resistance. This results in an imbalanced effect of ghrelin and leptin, which may lead to more weight gain and obesity.

- **Thyroid hormones – these manage and modulate metabolism**
  These are secreted by the thyroid gland in the neck and help manage metabolic processes and energy production. They are affected by lifestyle, including diet, nutrition, exercise (HIIT – high intensity interval training), stress and sleep. The thyroid responds to internal and external

factors and is one of the hormones responsible for metabolic adaptation when someone goes on a prolonged diet and exercise programme.

- **Adrenaline – known as the metabolic accelerator**
This is secreted by the adrenal gland and influences other hormones such as human growth hormone (HGH), cortisol and testosterone. The release of cortisol enhances its effects, however, prolonged release of adrenaline cannot be sustained and repeated stress results in exhaustion of adrenaline production, which then leaves behind an unbalanced release of cortisol.

Unopposed chronic cortisol release can lead to insulin resistance, metabolic syndrome, central body fat accumulation, muscle loss and bone matrix loss. There can also be immunosuppression, which can increase risk of infection, poor healing and even reduced surveillance against the chromosomal changes that result in cancer. Blood pressure and risk of heart disease can also increase.

- **Cortisol – known as the stress hormone**
This is secreted by the adrenal cortex. It has a beneficial effect in the acute stress response

in situations of fight, flight or freeze response in the presence of danger, when balanced with adrenaline. In the chronic situation it is not balanced with adrenaline and so has the detrimental effects discussed above.

- **Human Growth Hormone (HGH) – known as the 'anabolic' stimulator**
  This helps build muscle and burn fat at the same time. It works closely with adrenaline and cortisol to maintain vitality and youthfulness. These hormones are stimulated by HIIT (high intensity interval training) and Burst training (see also page 35) for less than thirty minutes at a time, maintaining a protein-adequate, balanced diet and getting plenty of sleep. Being sedentary, having poor sleep and eating a poorly balanced diet high in processed foods, as well as drinking excessive amounts of alcohol will damage the HGH production system.

  The production of HGH by the pituitary gland diminishes after the adolescent growth spurt and is only stimulated on demand after the mid-thirties as continuous levels of HGH in later life will accelerate the ageing process, disease processes and stimulate cancer cells.

- **Testosterone – known as the sculpting hormone** This is produced at higher levels in men than in women and gives them their muscular shape. It works in conjunction with oestrogen (higher levels in women than men) to maintain a healthy body.

  The male testosterone/oestrogen ratio results in a muscular 'V' shape, while the female testosterone/oestrogen ratio results in the hourglass shape. Testosterone stimulates receptors all over the body to influence a state of wellbeing, sex drive, lean body mass, bone density, muscular strength and energy levels. Enough exercise, sex and sleep help maintain healthy levels. A diet with sufficient good-quality protein will also help maintain healthy levels.

- **Oestrogen – known as the feminising hormone** This has a stronger influence on women, but is still present in men, though at lower levels. It is required to maintain a healthy lean body mass. To maintain appropriate levels of oestrogen, a healthy diet inclusive of healthy plant-based foods is necessary. Sufficient sleep and stress management is also important.

- **Progesterone – known as the friend of oestrogen** This works with oestrogen to give the female shape and works to reduce the negative effects of cortisol. Sufficient sleep and stress management will help maintain this hormone.

- **Incretins – Known as the food sensors**
  There are two of these in the body and they detect the ratio of food entering the small intestine and the relative amounts of fat, sugar, proteins and vegetable material entering the ilium:

1. GLP (glucagon-like peptide) is essentially a fat burner and sensitive to proteins and vegetables entering the small intestine.
2. GIP (glucose dependent insulinotropic – insulin-like – peptide) is a fat storer and sensitive to fat and sugars entering the small intestine.

- **Neuropeptide Y (NPY) – known as the fat amplifier**
  This is produced and secreted by the nerves of the sympathetic nervous system and in the brain. It causes growth and amplification of fat tissue. In childhood, it determines the number of fat cells in the body in response to the calorific intake. After the pre-adolescent phase, it works like cortisol in increasing food intake and fat storage.

- **Irisin – known as the exercise-related fat burner**
  This recently discovered hormone is secreted from muscle tissue after exercise. It increases fat burning and also improves cognitive function and feelings of general wellbeing. The most exciting effect of this hormone is that it appears to have an anti-ageing effect by lengthening telomeres, which can extend the life of cell lines, and so lengthen life expectancy and literally 'turn back time'. Evidence shows that exercising big muscle groups and, to a lesser extent, aerobic exercise, increases the secretion of this hormone.

- **MOTS-c – known as the Mitochondrial-Derived Peptide**
  This hormone works at the mitochondrial DNA level. It primarily targets muscle cells to modulate the mitochondrial DNA to promote metabolic homeostasis (balance). This in turn reduces obesity and insulin resistance. HIIT exercise on a regular basis (see also page 35) increases the number of mitochondria and so the effect of MOTS-c on the body.

HOW TO LOSE WEIGHT BY GETTING YOUR HUNGER HORMONES WORKING FOR YOU

1. **Avoid calorie restriction diets.** Prolonged calorie restriction increases ghrelin, reduces leptin and causes insulin and leptin resistance.

2. **Avoid processed foods.** These damage the metabolic system, causing insulin resistance, and also damage the leptin receptors.

3. **Eat enough good-quality protein.** This helps to control appetite and regulate ghrelin production. The recommended amount of protein is two portions per day. One portion is roughly the size and thickness of your palm for meat, fish and mycoprotein (such as Quorn), or two organic eggs.

4. **Exercise is also important, but what type of exercise is the most effective?** Historically, weight-loss advice was centred around low to moderate aerobic activity, such as walking, running, cycling or swimming. Research over the past ten years has actually shown that this type of exercise stimulates an increase in ghrelin and a reduction in leptin production, thereby

stimulating hunger and increasing appetite. Prolonged aerobic exercise has also been shown to reduce testosterone levels. The initial increase in metabolism appears to stop after three months as a result of 'metabolic adaptation' and we hit a 'wall' with respect to weight loss; weight then starts to increase again, despite exercising. Prolonged aerobic exercise has also been shown to increase levels of cortisol. Research has shown that there are two types of exercise that (a) burn abdominal fat and control appetite and hunger, and (b) control weight gain in the short and long term. These are:

- **'Burst training'**. This involves exertion at 90 per cent of your maximum for thirty seconds for five sets, three times a week. Exercise intensely for thirty seconds then rest for forty seconds, before repeating the exercise. During the rest period, it is best to keep moving and not to sit down. You should be able to complete this in 10 to 15 minutes per session.

- **'High-intensity interval training' (HIIT)**. This has been shown to be the most effective exercise for reducing hunger and appetite, and controlling weight in both the long and short term.

It is important to note that metabolic adaptation can decrease the efficiency of any exercise, so it is important to change the exercises every three months. There is also evidence to show that exercising first thing on an empty stomach gives the greatest benefits with respect to improving glucose tolerance and ghrelin/leptin balance.

5. **A good night's sleep (seven to nine hours)**. Sleep deprivation has been shown to be associated with poor ghrelin/leptin balance. Good-quality sleep has been shown to better regulate appetite and the desire to eat unhealthy snacks in comparison to exercising later in the day, after eating.

6. **Reducing and managing stress** has been shown to result in a favourable ghrelin/leptin balance, and so weight management. Chronic stress results in raised cortisol levels, which has a negative effect on metabolism, ghrelin/leptin balance, and can result in insulin resistance. Finding the time for meditation, mindfulness and relaxation is important.

7. **Avoid high glycaemic index (GI) foods** (these are foods, namely carbohydrates, that release sugar very quickly into the blood supply), and

those high in sugar and artificial sweeteners. These include:

- cakes, biscuits, cookies, pastries and other sweets, chocolate and ice cream
- fizzy drinks and drinks with a high sugar content
- pizza, white bread, pita, rolls and wraps
- salted snacks like crisps
- foods fried at high temperatures

In conclusion, there are lots of weight-loss systems and clinics out there. Some are more scientific than others, but they all present us with a system, and some even prescribe slimming pills, which can be very dangerous (in that they are based on stimulators, such as amphetamines, which can have adverse effects on your heart and can cause psychological problems). Research has shown that none of the previously used systems actually work and that most people will regain the initial weight they lose because the systems are not sustainable as a normal lifestyle.

Despite billions spent each year on weight-loss programmes, the incidence of obesity, metabolic disease (such as type 2 diabetes) and environmentally determined diseases continues to rise. My hope is that this book will serve to educate and guide you to making informed and intelligent changes to your lifestyle in order to 'turn back time' and still continue to enjoy a long, healthy and happy life.

CHAPTER 3

HORMONAL IMPACT ON FAT DISTRIBUTION AND AGEING

Most imbalances in the body are due to inflammation, which in turn, affects hormonal imbalances.

BODY FAT STORAGE SITE	HORMONE IMBALANCE
Belly	High cortisol/high insulin/high testosterone/ low or high oestrogen
Hips (butt and hamstring)	High oestrogen
Triceps	High insulin/low DHEA (Dehydroepiandrosterone, a steroid based hormone produced by the adrenal glands and the brain. It is involved in the synthesis of androgenic hormones, and in metabolism)
Love handles	High insulin
Chest	High oestrogen
Back	High insulin/low thyroid
Thighs	Low growth hormone

CORTISOL

Cortisol is a 'master' hormone produced by the adrenal cortex (the outer part of the adrenal gland that produces hormones, including stress hormones) and is released in response to chronic or repeated stress and low blood glucose concentrations. Its function in the body is to increase blood sugar through gluconeogenesis (by metabolising proteins into sugar) to suppress the immune system; it also decreases bone formation, diverting the process into gluconeogenesis in favour of osteogenesis (bone formation).

It is also activated in fasting, and calorie restriction, especially carbohydrate restriction. This is one of the body's protective responses to possible starvation.

Chronic release of cortisol will eventually lead to chronic rises in blood glucose with overstimulation of insulin production and the eventual development of glucose intolerance, insulin resistance, beta cell (the cells that produce insulin) exhaustion, and, ultimately, can lead to diabetes. Prolonged periods of raised cortisol results in muscle loss, increase in belly fat, suppression of the immune system with increased risk of infections, thinning of the skin and premature ageing, osteoporosis and bone fractures, fragility of blood vessels, high blood pressure, heart disease and an increased risk of cancer through weakening the T-cell and natural killer cells (these are part of the immune system that look for early changes in cells that may lead to cancer, and destroy them).

Cortisol also inhibits collagen and elastin production, thereby weakening the infrastructure of skin, bones, blood vessels and all of the tissues in the body; it slows down and inhibits wound healing; and it has an effect on the kidneys by increasing sodium retention and potassium excretion, which can result in high blood pressure. Cortisol increases the gastric excretions, and decreases the gastric defences, thereby increasing the risk of gastric and duodenal ulcers and bleeding. Changes in the normal daily patterns of cortisol can lead to sleep disorders, mood and anxiety disorders, and depressive disorders. Chronic cortisol elevation can also decrease fertility.

High cortisol also interferes with thyroid function, and can lead to an underactive thyroid response. The body shape changes to resemble a 'lemon on sticks' as a result of muscle loss in the arms and legs, and excess belly fat.

A 24-hour saliva test to assess your personal levels of stress and adrenal fatigue may be useful if you're concerned (unfortunately this is not available on the NHS, and has to be arranged privately). Fortunately, your cortisol levels can be managed using meditation, supplementation, nutrition and exercise.

CORTISOL BALANCING RECOMMENDATIONS

Foods to choose:

- Have two dates and five almonds within thirty minutes of getting up in the morning.
- Consume brown basmati rice and oatmeal, which are soothing to the nerves.
- Choose foods that are rich in magnesium, such as apricot, banana, cantaloupe melons, seafood, organic soybeans, kelp, lima beans and avocado. Having a bath in Epsom salts will also increase the magnesium uptake through your skin.
- Eat raw, fresh vegetables and fruits for their vitamin, mineral, fibre and enzyme content.
- Consume foods high in tryptophan (a precursor to serotonin which is important for sleep, and general mood), such as organic eggs, dairy and turkey, fish, brown rice and nut butters.
- B3 is beneficial for the nervous system and general energy release in cells. This can be found in wholegrains, poultry, figs, dates and dried legumes.
- Vitamin B6 is good for the nervous system and general energy release, and stabilises metabolism. This is found in lentils, oats, peas, raw sunflower

seeds, plantains, grapes, kiwi, cabbage, peppers and carrots.

- Include chamomile, skullcap and peppermint teas in your diet, which support the nervous system and help to reduce stress and hence cortisol production.

Foods to avoid:

- Excessive caffeine activates the sympathetic nervous system and drains the body of B vitamins, making you feel nervous and jumpy. Try to restrict this to less than three cups a day, and not after 6pm. Some people are not genetically sensitive to caffeine, while others are. This can be seen in your genetic profiling.
- Chemical additives in food upset the neurological and hormonal and chemical functioning of your body, so try to consume single-ingredient foods, i.e. those that are recognisable as what they should be and have not been processed and added to. Remember to always read the ingredients on the packaging.
- Alcohol is a mood depressor that can trigger hypoglycaemic symptoms and lead to feelings of anxiety. It is also a cellular toxin, especially

to liver cells. Moderate amounts of alcohol have been shown to be of benefit and have a protective effect. Excess alcohol can inhibit the liver's ability to mobilise free fatty acids and so prevent fat loss. The liver is also our most powerful detoxifying organ, so if it is being inhibited, other toxins will build up in our system, causing further metabolic and hormonal upset, as well as build-up of certain medical drugs to a toxic level. Your sensitivity to alcohol, again, can be shown in your genetic profile.

- Excess sugar causes hyperglycaemia and anxiety and can make you feel restless, tired and depressed. It also robs the body of B vitamins. Sugar is highly toxic and is rapidly eliminated from the circulation because it is highly reactive and toxic to cells and the components of your body. Prolonged high levels of blood sugar interact with the amino acids in your proteins to form 'Advanced End Glycation Products', which then act as free radicals, causing damage to the rest of the cells of the body, and to collagen and elastin that make up the intracellular structure. Our bodies require sugar for metabolism, however, it is also toxic at high levels. Consumption of low GI carbs is therefore important. This allows a slow and steady release of glucose, which can be metabolised effectively without it peeking into toxic levels.

- Excess table salt (more than five grams per day or one teaspoon) can cause a sodium/potassium imbalance. The mineral potassium is important for the normal function of the nervous system, the heart, and the stability of the cell membranes of all the cells of the body.
- Processed, refined junk foods deplete the body of nutrients, especially B vitamins and minerals, which are important for a properly functioning nervous system. They also contain hormones, preservatives and other chemicals that interfere with the normal and healthy functioning of our bodies. Usually they contain very high levels of sugar. Aim to have single-ingredient foods in their basic form and avoid processed foods.
- Be sure to exercise regularly, but not before bedtime.
- Reduce stress through meditation, mindfulness and reading.
- Avoid high calories in the form of sugars and high GI carbohydrates in late-night meals.
- If you are hungry late at night, some nuts, cherries or a slice of chicken breast meat will help stave

off the hunger and help you get a good night's sleep.

- Avoid looking at blue light last thing at night (this includes devices such as the television and other electronic devices, including electronic books) as this mimics daylight and can interfere with sleep.

OESTROGEN

Oestrogen balancing recommendations

Foods to eat:

- Foods high in B vitamins (especially B6, also known as pyridoxine). These foods aid in reducing the symptoms of premenstrual syndrome (PMS) such as water retention, irritability and fatigue. PMS can also cause symptoms such as confusion and muscle pains and worsen the symptoms of any pre-existing anaemia and deterioration of vision. Include foods such as tuna, turkey and chicken breast, grass-fed beef, lentils, pinto beans, oats, rye, wheat germ, spinach, avocados, millet, carrots and pistachio nuts in your diet.
- Foods high in fibre, such as beans, chickpeas, spelt, millet, dried peas, flax seed, brown rice,

barley, oat bran, wild brown and black rice and oats. The fibre in these foods will help to eliminate toxins from the body. There are two types of fibre in our diet:

1. Soluble fibre (found in plant cells), which includes pectins, gum and mucilage. Its role is to lower levels of LDL (low density lipoprotein) cholesterol, which is generally known to be the 'bad boy' cholesterol. This can also help with constipation. Examples of foods rich in this type of fibre include fruits and vegetables, beans, peas and lentils.
2. Insoluble fibre (which makes up the structural parts of the plant cell walls). This includes cellulose, hemicellulose and lignin. Its role is to add bulk to the faeces. This helps prevent constipation, piles and diverticular disease. Examples of foods rich in this type of fibre include unrefined wheat bran, corn bran, rice bran, the skins of fruit and vegetables, wholegrain foods, nuts and seeds.

There is also good evidence that a healthy combination of both types of fibres helps reduce the risk of heart and bowel diseases, including cancer. It is recommended that adults should consume twenty-five to thirty grams of fibre daily.

- Resistant starch is the starch that is resistant to digestion in the small bowel and so it passes to the large bowel, where the bacteria ferment and change it to short-chain fatty acids, which also help lower cholesterol and reduce bowel cancer. It is found in unprocessed grains and cereals, potatoes, lentils and unripe bananas. Fermented vegetables, such as sauerkraut provide us with high levels of these short-chain fatty acids and so provide a health benefit.

- Include fresh raw, organic fruits and vegetables for their vitamin, mineral and enzyme content. These tend to go off quickly because of the presence of enzymes. Non-organic fruits and vegetables may have a much longer shelf life, but may not provide us with the same levels of useable vitamins and minerals.

- Be sure to use unrefined, cold-pressed oils that contain omega-3 and omega-6 essential fatty acids. The ratio of these should be 1:1 in order to get the best health benefits. High levels of omega-6, as found in the modern diet, can lead to inflammation in the body. Most vegetable oils are high in omega-6, which can cause inflammation. Flaxseed and fish oils are richer in omega-3 oils. Omega-3 is also high in grass-fed meats as it is in chia seeds. Higher ratios of omega-3 and omega-6 have been shown to be protective against diseases such as heart disease, type 2 diabetes, obesity, metabolic syndrome, IBS and inflammatory bowel disease, macular degeneration, inflammatory arthritis, asthma, cancer, psychiatric disorders and autoimmune disease. There is evidence that a high omega-6:omega-3 ratio is detrimental to certain genetic variations that can increase risk of atherosclerosis (a disease in which plaque builds up in the arteries) and heart disease.

- Vitamin E is a potent antioxidant that reduces free radical damage and slows down the environmental ageing process. It helps to reduce cholesterol levels (thereby protecting against heart disease), helps repair damaged skin by speeding up cellular regeneration (thereby acting as a natural anti-ageing nutrient) and also helps protect against cigarette smoke and ultraviolet- induced free radical damage (thereby protecting against skin and other cancers). When combined with vitamin C it helps to reduce inflammation (thereby helpful in the treatment of sunburn, acne, eczema and the treatment of healing scars); it also helps thicken hair and reduces dryness and scaling of the scalp; it helps to balance hormones and maintain weight, and improves circulation. It may also help to relieve breast tenderness and ease the symptoms of PMS.

When combined with vitamin C, beta-carotene and zinc, vitamin E helps to protect against and improves macular degeneration. It helps protect against age-related dementia and also Alzheimer's disease. Research has shown that it may help reduce cancer and improve the effects of treating cancer through its powerful antioxidant effect. Vitamin E can improve post-exercise recovery and improve endurance and muscle strength. It also helps to reduce bruising in the elderly by improving the strength of capillary walls.

Vitamin E plays an essential role in the neurological and brain development of the baby in the first 1,000 following conception (that is up to the age of two years).

Foods that are rich in vitamin E include vegetables, such as spinach and broccoli; cereals, such as wheat germ and oatmeal; roots, such as sweet potato; fruits, such as blueberries, kiwi, mango, avocados, tomatoes and butternut squash; nuts, such as almonds and hazelnuts; and raw sunflower seeds.

There are eight major forms of vitamin E, some more active than others (alpha and beta the least active, delta and gamma the most active), and all forms being essential in a balanced diet. Research has shown that high levels of Alpha-tocotrienol may interfere with the absorption of other forms and it is this form that is usually present in most of the supplements. It is, therefore, better to get our dietary intake of vitamin E through a healthy, balanced diet.

- Magnesium and calcium are helpful in relieving symptoms such as nervousness, cramping and irritability, and can be found in foods such as avocados, cantaloupe melon, seafood, bananas, brown rice, raw almonds and pumpkin seeds.

- Drink plenty of bottled spring water (preferably from glass and not plastic bottles), unsweetened fresh juices (it is always better to have the whole fruit rather than the juice as your sugar intake is higher with juices, and you may miss out on a lot of the fibre and other vitamins and minerals) and herbal teas.

- Follow a regular exercise plan to help circulation and the elimination of toxins. Exercise may also aid in reducing cramps due to menstruation. Avoid smoking and, where possible, reduce stress in your life.

- Where possible, choose foods that are organic

as non-organic foods may contain unwanted hormones and chemicals.

Foods to avoid:

- Alcohol – due to its high sugar content and tendency towards nutrient deficiencies and cellular toxicity.
- Dairy products like milk and cream cheese as these can be high in lactose, the milk sugar that we find difficult to digest after the age of four years. Kefir (a fermented milk drink) and certain live yogurts are good for your gut and general health.
- Saturated fat as found in red meat (except for grass-fed beef), sausages, cold cuts and bacon.
- Foods containing high sodium, canned foods, fast foods and junk foods. Sodium causes water retention and the excretion of calcium. Sea salt in moderation, however, is good for your health.
- All sweets and sugars – they will rob the body of nutrients and stress your metabolism.
- Caffeine – as found in black tea, chocolate, colas and coffee. Caffeine has a diuretic effect that can cause mineral depletion when taken in large

amounts. Some people are genetically more sensitive to caffeine.

- Tap water may contain high levels of oestrogen.
- Avoid taking birth control pills if possible.

THYROID

Thyroid balancing recommendations

Foods to eat:

- Organic, fermented dairy products such as natural unsweetened yogurt or kefir with live cultures.
- Zinc-containing foods that boost the immune system such as raw sunflower and pumpkin seeds, nuts, mushrooms, chickpeas and lentils.
- Iodine is good for the thyroid, especially when combined with selenium. Choose foods that are rich in iodine, such as saltwater fish, sesame seeds, seafood, kelp, Nova Scotia dulse seaweed, asparagus and sea salt.
- Eat lots of fresh, raw fruits and vegetables.
- Foods high in B vitamins, like organic brown rice, oats, rye, wheat germ and molasses. B vitamins impart a benefit upon immune function and stress.

- In addition, be sure to perform daily exercise to improve circulation.

Foods to avoid:

- Processed and frozen ready-made foods. White flour and white rice products that are lacking in nutrients.

- All fried foods.

- Avoid excessive fluoride and chlorine found in tap water and toothpaste – they can block iodine receptions in the thyroid gland. Cooking with tap water or drinking it after boiling is not so bad as the chlorine will evaporate, reducing the levels. It is important to appreciate that fluoride in toothpaste is important for dental health, and the small amounts that are effective and present do not pose a risk to health, as far as evidence is concerned. Note that fluoride toothpaste should only be introduced after the age of 3 years in children.

- Hydrogenated oils, margarine and shortening (or vegetable oil dripping).

- Sugars, artificial sweeteners and sweets can weaken the immune system and may lead to auto-immune conditions of the thyroid.

- Consume these foods in moderation: broccoli, Brussels sprouts, cabbage, mustard greens, kale, peaches, pears, radishes, spinach and turnips. Known as goitrogenic foods, they may further suppress thyroid function.

TESTOSTERONE

Testosterone balancing recommendations

Foods to eat:

- Dandelion greens and parsley.
- Vitamin E containing foods such as soy beans, cornmeal, unrefined oils, Nova Scotia dulse seaweed, wheat germ and dark leafy green vegetables. These foods and their vitamin E content are excellent for the circulatory system and act as an antioxidant.
- Fresh fruits and vegetables for their high vitamin, mineral, enzyme and fibre content.
- Foods that are high in zinc and essential fatty acids such as raw unsalted nuts and seeds, including pumpkin and sunflower, organic eggs, fish, seafood, sardines and dried legumes.
- Wholegrain cereals and breads, organic brown

rice, kamut grain, (a protein, and fatty acids, rich Khorasan wheat grain, that is gaining popularity, and is available in health food shops or sections of the supermarkets. oats and spelt.

Unrefined cold-pressed flax seed oil, walnut oil and fish oils high in omega-3 fatty acids.

- Foods high in selenium such as tuna, mackerel, Brazil nuts, wholegrains, garlic and onions.
- Vegetarians can enjoy fermented organic soy such as tofu and miso.
- Be sure to participate in a regular fitness programme of both cardiovascular and resistance training. Practice relaxation techniques, avoid smoking and second-hand smoke inhalation.

Foods to avoid:

- Processed foods such as instant and pre-prepared fast foods.
- All white flour products, including white bread, white rice, pasta, buns, pita, etc.
- Hydrogenated oils, shortening, butter substitutes and margarine.
- Carbonated drinks, tap water and excessive alcohol.

- Artificial ingredients such as preservatives, additives, artificial colour, sweeteners and flavourings.
- Excessive amounts of caffeine (keep it under three single shots per day).
- Sugar and sweets.
- Pesticides – be sure to clean all fruit and vegetables thoroughly.
- Fast-grown meats containing hormones and antibiotics (livestock matures over a longer period if it is naturally grass fed. To grow and mature cattle more quickly they are fed on grains and corn, and other types of artificial feeds, and may be stimulated with growth and sex hormones in order to accelerate the maturation process. One of the problems of feeding ruminators, i.e. animals with two stomach chambers like cows, is that they develop obstructions and infections, which then require antibiotics and other drugs. These build up in the animals, and enter our food chain when we consume them) .

CHAPTER 4

THE MENOPAUSE

The menopause (also known as 'the change of life' or simply 'the change') refers to that time in every woman's life when her periods stop and her ovaries lose their reproductive function and their ability to secrete the hormones oestrogen and progesterone. Usually, this occurs between the ages of forty-five and fifty-five. In the UK the average age is fifty-one. In rare cases women may become menopausal in their thirties, or even younger. This is then known as a premature menopause, or premature ovarian insufficiency or failure.

The effects of the menopause reflect the change in the balance of hormones where there is a reproduction of oestrogens in comparison to testosterone.

SIGNS AND SYMPTOMS

The loss of reproductive function can have a psychological effect that may be very distressing and require further help from a GP. Hot flushes and night sweats are common symptoms, occurring in about 75 per cent of women. These commonly occur in the first year after the last period. Other symptoms include sleeplessness, restless legs syndrome, vaginal dryness, skin dryness and irritation, skin sensitivity, thinning out and weakness of the pelvic structures resulting in urinary frequency, stress incontinence and increased risk of urinary infections, as well as dyspareunia (painful sexual intercourse).

The mental and psychological changes include loss of sex drive, anxiousness, low mood, poor sleep and even depression. Other features can be seen as forgetfulness, with poor memory and recall. All of this can lead to loss of confidence, and even social avoidance and isolation. In many women this is also the time when their children have grown up and are leaving home, the 'empty nest syndrome', which may also contribute to the psychological state of mind.

Physical changes after the menopause include loss of bone volume and osteoporosis. Then there are metabolic changes that increase fat deposition around the abdomen, which can further contribute to loss of confidence. Physiological changes with insulin resistance, raised cholesterol, and triglycerides and raised blood pressure can all lead to an increased risk of heart disease and stroke.

Skin changes are also seen. Oestrogen is an inhibitor of the action of collagenase, the enzyme that breaks down collagen. This means that collagenase becomes more active once oestrogen declines. This, combined with reduced cellular activity and reduced collagen production, leads to the accelerated appearance of the signs of ageing and thinning of the skin. A healthy oestrogen and testosterone balance before menopause helps regulate inflammation in the body. Following menopause, the inflammatory factors increase. This leads to more aches and pains, and in the skin results in increased sensitivity, and can even result in redness, flushing, and broken blood vessels, and increased bruising. The skin can also become dry and itchy.

An imbalance between oestrogenising and androgenising hormones in favour of testosterone results in loss of pinkness of the skin, especially the lips, a coarsening of the skin and features, growth of facial hair and even the appearance of acne. There can also be thinning of scalp hair. The best way to combat these changes is to look at your diet, nutrition, exercise and skincare.

TREATING THE MENOPAUSE

The menopause is a natural part of ageing, and so is not a disease process or a condition that requires treatment. It is important not to medicalise this process. As many women experience symptoms of the change in hormonal balance, these can be supported and the risk factors managed. That being said, many women go through the menopause without any intervention whatsoever. There is a change in the risk profile of all postmenopausal women, which should be managed and reduced but this can be done with diet, good nutrition and exercise. Hormonal support and balancing can also be of benefit with respect to symptoms, physical and physiological changes, and risk control.

Blood tests can also show your doctor the hormonal imbalance, so he, or she can correct it with hormone replacement therapy (HRT), both medically and with natural bio-identical hormones. However, there can be side effects to the hormonal treatments, if not balanced properly, such as weight gain, tender breasts, water retention, migraines, depression and sickness. It is recommended that HRT be used only to control the short-term menopausal symptoms for up to three years as long-term use has been linked with an increased risk of breast cancer and thrombosis. Long-term hormonal balancing can be useful to reduce the risks associated with the menopause, while at the same time reducing the risks associated with full HRT.

Part of the 'Female Ageing Syndrome' is characterised by other hormonal changes, such as diminishing testosterone and thyroid function. There is also a change in the absorption of and levels of iron, vitamin B12 and vitamin D levels. There appear to be associated changes in the levels of serotonin and dopamine too. Skincare that contains peptides and stem cell factors also acts like bio-identical, or bio-mimetic hormone replacement for your skin, keeping it healthy and youthful.

OPTIMAL DIET FOR THE MENOPAUSE

There has been a lot of research into what would be a good diet to reduce menopausal symptoms and help prevent the physical and physiological changes and risks associated with the menopause. It is important to implement this type of diet early, before the onset of the change, in order to get the most benefit. In fact, I would recommend that the basic principles be implemented from the mid-thirties, 'The Tipping Point' (see also page 15).

Water

Good hydration with healthy mineral water from glass bottles is the best way of maintaining an optimal cellular environment for healthy hormonal and physiological activity. Remember, 5 per cent dehydration = 20 per cent loss of efficiency.

Calcium and magnesium

We know that calcium is essential for bone health. However, research also shows it may help protect against cancer, diabetes and heart disease, and manage blood pressure. It also supports nerve and muscle function, helps with weight loss, maintains dental health and helps prevent symptoms of Premenstrual Syndrome (PMS). Calcium is involved with the control of the levels of potassium, phosphorous and magnesium in the body.

We must remember that magnesium is essential for the absorption of calcium, so foods rich in both are essential. Calcium supplements by themselves may not be absorbed sufficiently. Getting calcium from a healthy diet is the best way of supplementation. Foods rich in calcium and magnesium are:

- whey protein
- sardines
- kefir (a fermented milk drink)
- raw milk (milk that has not been pasteurised). This is safe if sourced from reputable, trusted sources, who have reared and tested the animals, like eggs are now safe to have raw. These should

be avoided, as should all raw dairy produce during pregnancy, nursing, and in young children

- white beans
- unpasteurised milk cheese, this again is safe if sourced from trusted sources
- kidney beans
- sesame seeds
- okra
- collard greens – these are certain loose-leafed brassica group of vegetables such as cabbage, broccoli, kale and spring greens.
- almonds
- natto (Japanese fermented soy beans)
- goat cheese
- mustard greens

Vitamin D

Essential, not just for good bone health, but also healthy immune and hormonal systems, cardiovascular system, neurological and muscular systems, skin health and tendons. Sources of vitamin D include:

- sunlight: aim for ten to twenty minutes of unexposed sun per day. This may vary with skin pigmentation and where in the world you are
- halibut
- carp

- mackerel
- eel
- maitake mushrooms
- salmon
- whitefish
- portobello mushrooms
- swordfish
- rainbow trout
- cod liver oil
- sardines
- tuna
- organic, free-range chicken eggs
- raw milk

Fruit and vegetables

These help stabilise the metabolism and provide a good source of antioxidants, which help maintain a healthy weight. Eating fresh, organic, non-GM, whole and seasonal fruit and vegetables is the best way to get your essential vitamins and minerals as they are contained in synergistic combinations with the enzymes required for optimal absorption. It is amazing how good nature is at designing our multivitamin and mineral supplements.

Foods rich in vitamin B

Eating foods rich in vitamin B complexes can help boost energy, calm stress and maintain a healthy digestive system. Vitamin B1 (thiamine) examples of foods include:

- nutritional yeast
- seaweed
- sunflower seeds
- macadamia nuts
- black beans
- lentils
- beef liver – it is important to remember that the amount of meat we consume should reduce with age, especially over 50 years of age. We require half the amount we did in our 30s
- asparagus
- brussels sprouts

This helps maintain a healthy metabolism, nervous, cardiovascular and immune systems. B1 is also used in the treatment of alcoholism and dementia. It has a positive effect on mood and age-related vision deterioration, especially night vision.

Vitamin B2 (Riboflavin) examples of foods include:

- healthy organic grass-fed meat and offal
- seaweed
- mollusks

- mackerel
- organic free-range chicken eggs
- organic dairy cheeses
- green leafy vegetables
- beans and legumes
- almonds and seeds
- tahini

This helps prevent migraines, supports vision, maintains energy levels and has an antioxidant effect, helping protect against free radical damage. It is also important for healthy hair and skin, and is used to treat and prevent anaemia.

Vitamin B3 (niacin/niacinamide), examples of foods include:

- organic grass-fed beef liver and steak
- organic, free-range chicken breasts
- organic wild tuna
- sunflower seeds
- organic grass-fed lamb
- organic wild salmon
- sardines
- turkey

B3 helps maintain cardiovascular health and metabolism. It is essential for healthy brain function, healthy skin and regulates metabolism; it may help to control, and even prevent, diabetes. It is best taken as part of a healthy diet as supplements can cause side effects such as nausea, vomiting, headaches, dizziness, gastric upset with ulcers, low blood pressure and fainting, to list but a few.

Vitamin B5 (pantothenic acid) examples of foods include:

- organic grass-fed beef liver
- avocados
- sunflower seeds
- organic free-range duck
- portobello mushrooms
- organic free-range chicken eggs
- organic wild salmon
- lentils
- broccoli

This is involved in the release of energy and metabolic balancing; also balancing cholesterol, controlling blood pressure and protection against heart disease. B5 improves neurotransmission in the brain and peripheral nervous system. Also involved in maintaining a healthy gut and immune system, it enhances the effects of the other B vitamins in a synergistic way. It plays an important part in the manufacture of sex- and stress-related hormones. The beneficial effects of vitamin B5 are that it helps reduce fatigue, irritability, depression, anxiety, insomnia, stomach pains, nausea and vomiting, burning feet, restless legs, muscle cramps and respiratory infections.

Vitamin B6 (Pyridoxine), examples of foods include:

- organic free-range turkey breasts
- organic grass-fed beef
- pistachio nuts
- organic wild tuna
- pinto beans
- avocados
- organic free-range chicken breasts
- sunflower seeds
- sesame seeds

B6 is involved in maintaining a healthy metabolic system, neurological system, immune system and liver function. It also helps maintain healthy skin and eyes and is involved with red blood cell manufacture and the production of antibodies. It has a role in pain management and elevates mood.

Vitamin B12 examples of foods include:

- organic grass-fed beef liver, also high in iron and folic acid

- sardines, also high in omega-3 fatty acids
- wild Atlantic mackerel, also high in omega-3 fatty acids, and coming from the Atlantic, it is low in mercury content and is rated for sustainability
- organic grass-fed lamb, also rich in protein, iron, selenium and zinc
- organic wild salmon is also particularly rich in vitamin D
- nutritional yeast also contains nine of the eighteen essential amino acids (those that humans cannot manufacture)
- feta cheese, also rich in vitamin B12
- organic grass-fed beef, also high in antioxidants and building blocks for vitamins A and E
- cottage cheese, also a good source of protein and calcium
- organic free-range chicken eggs also contain liver-supporting choline

The benefits of vitamin B12 include:

- helps maintain energy
- provides neurological protection, including against dementia and Alzheimer's disease
- boosts mood and prevents depression and anxiety; also helps with dealing with stress

- gives healthy skin and hair
- maintains a healthy cardiovascular and digestive system
- provides protection against certain types of cancer
- is involved in the production of healthy red blood cells.

Iron

The requirement for iron actually goes down after the menopause, as there is no more menstrual bleeding. Iron supplementation after the menopause is not, therefore, recommended, as it can quickly build up and cause problems of iron overload.

CHAPTER 5

TACKLING DIET AND NUTRITION, AND THE IMPORTANCE OF THE GUT

'You are what you eat' is a common phrase that refers to the notion that to be fit, you need to eat good food. This phrase is derived from an article written by Jean Anthelme Brillat-Savarin in 1826, which translates to 'Tell me what you eat and I will tell you what you are'. Later, in 1863, Ludwig Andreas Feuerbach wrote in an essay, 'man is what he eats'.

Throughout history the notion of good nutrition has been linked to enjoying good health. Societies have offered sacrifice in the hope of receiving a good harvest of crops, or a good catch. In 1549, Archbishop Thomas Cranmer wrote the following prayer:

> 'We offer and present unto thee, O Lord, ourselves, our souls and bodies, to be a reasonable, holy, and living sacrifice unto thee; humbly beseeching thee that we, and all others who shall be partakers of this Holy Communion, may worthily receive the most precious Body and Blood of thy Son Jesus Christ, be filled by thy grace and heavenly benediction, and made one body with him, that he may dwell in us and we in him.'

For as long as history shows, food has been central to how communities have developed and survived. In poorer communities there appears to be a real fear of starvation, and being overweight is thought of as being healthy and associated with prosperity. It is unfortunate that as the population of the world has grown, the need to feed them has also become more urgent. Farming and scientific techniques to manipulate food have progressed to a point where not only has the nutritional value of food started to suffer, but some of the processed foods that are now available are harmful to our health. The phrase 'You are no longer what you eat, but are what your food eats' is becoming a more appropriate description of the modern diet.

WHAT ARE THE RISKS OF TODAY'S FOOD?

There is a lot of confusion about what to eat and what to avoid from a health risk perspective. I hope that this chapter will help to clarify some of the issues.

General use of pesticides

These are used to kill weeds (herbicides), insects (insecticides), fungus (fungicides), rodents (rodenticides) and others in order to increase crop yield.

These chemicals that are designed to kill cellular structures are released into our environment and can be introduced into our systems via food, water and air. Some pesticides have been shown to be so harmful that they have been banned.

The GMO (genetically modified organism) debate

This refers to genetic modification of plants to protect them against disease or damage from pests, and to survive environmental stress, such as droughts or floods.

Plant modification through cross-breeding, or hybridisation has been used for centuries in order to produce more robust crops. However, this can take years to achieve the results so methods of genetic modification have been developed to achieve this more specifically and quickly. This technology was first applied in the mid-1980s. The risk of toxicity and genetic transference has been discussed. However, years of studies have shown that there are little or no risks to health. The transgenesis of plants is not the problem: the problem may be with the monopoly that the companies who develop GMO crops may create, and the eventual loss of variety of food available to us. There may also be an environmental issue of nonspecific harm to useful insects like bees and butterflies from the insecticide effect in the crops. This may have a knock-on effect of loss of insect-eating bird population from the environment, and so on.

So, GMO crops do not pose a health risk to humans at present. However, there is a potential risk of them being controlled, monopolised and even weaponised as some of our gut bacteria produce plasmid (a special genetic structure in a cell that can replicate independently of the chromosomes. It acts like a machine that can introduce new genetic material into the organism. In bacteria they carry genetic information like antibiotic resistance, that can serve to protect the bacteria), which can transfer genetic material, such as antibiotic resistance to other bacteria, and possibly our gut cells. Some GMO modifications reduce the amount of natural enzymes that the plants have, and so extend shelf life. This can result in fewer nutrients being available for us to absorb.

For the sake of variety, while natural seasonal products are still available, I prefer to go organic, seasonal and

GMO-free. This is a personal choice, and not because of any proven risk from GMO crops at present.

The livestock debate

Healthy meat comes from healthy livestock, and healthy livestock comes from natural organic environments.

It is important to ensure that the fish, poultry and meat we consume is from healthy livestock sources and we don't overconsume. Remember that the right portion is the size and thickness of your palm (or a deck of cards), or about 75g. Ensure that the fish is caught in deep seas, so it is free of heavy metal and pesticide contamination. Also, that the meat and poultry is field reared and grass-fed, and that the eggs are from field reared poultry. This type of rearing does not require antibiotics or intervention to treat problems that forced reared animals experience. Such animals also have high stress levels and may be treated with hormones to speed up their growth. Minimise your intake of smoked or cured meats. Aim to totally cut out processed foods – these are high in potentially harmful additives and preservatives, which increase your free radical load.

The GI carbs debate

It is well-known that low GI carbohydrates are much better for your metabolism than the high GI carbohydrates. This, simply put, means that you should eat unprocessed carbohydrates in their simplest, naturally recognisable form.

Colourful fruit and vegetables are better than white starchy ones. Those that are in season are nutritionally better as they have not been in cold storage for lengthy periods of time. Organically grown fruit and vegetables are not exposed to pesticides and may have a shorter shelf life, but I believe they are tastier and better for you.

The healthy fats debate

For years there has been a debate about which are the healthiest fats. The answer is simple: 'All fats from healthy animals (grass-fed livestock) and healthy plants (cold-pressed, and not modified through hydrogenation) are healthy in moderation.

When cooking with any fat or oil, it is important to remember not to heat it to smoking point and not to keep on using the same oil for repeated frying, as free radicals can build up over time. A healthy amount of fat or oil is about two tablespoons a day per person on average.

Remember, everything in moderation: a little of what you like is good for you.

The debate about spicing things up

There is nothing worse than eating tasteless, bland food, so spicing things up doesn't just make things more pleasurable, but the herbs and spices can also have a beneficial effect on health and wellness.

Many herbs and spices have been used for their medicinal properties in the past and there is much medical evidence about their effects in treating diseases and conditions. The only thing to be careful about is not to have too much salt as sodium chloride can affect the cardiovascular system and the kidneys. Sea salt and Himalayan salt appear to be the best to use as they contain a complex of minerals that are good for health. It is also important to remember to balance the other minerals such as magnesium and selenium for optimal health.

The debate about water and wine

It is important to remain well hydrated as most of the bodily reactions occur in an aqueous environment. If you are 5 per cent dehydrated then the efficiency of your body is reduced by 20 per cent.

It is also important to realise that you will not feel thirsty until you are 15 per cent dehydrated, so it is important to drink small amounts of water regularly throughout the day. I would recommend a glassful (175ml) every hour and remember that if you have a caffeinated drink, you need to replace the water you lose with twice the volume of water.

The debate about when and how to eat

Should we have three meals a day, or is it better to graze? Breakfast or not? Should we eat before exercise, or after it? These are complex questions and everyone is different in their requirements depending on lifestyle, exercise routines and genetic requirements.

The simple advice I would give is not to restrict your calorie intake for long periods of time, or to regularly fast. Try to eat foods that are recognisable. I would recommend that you buy single food items rather than pre-prepared processed foods. Don't wait to eat until you are starving as you can overeat. Take your time when eating and enjoy the smells and flavours of your food, chewing each mouthful at least twenty times before swallowing, as this prepares your digestive system to receive your food and get the most out of it. I would also advise that you do not drink too much water during meals as it can dilute the enzymes that are working on your ingested food.

Eating should be a pleasurable experience and your diet should be enjoyable, something to look forward to, and sustainable. This will also serve to relieve stress and anxiety, and help maintain a healthy psychological and mental state.

CHAPTER 6

EXERCISE: PRACTICAL EXERCISES AND HOW TO DO THEM

There's an exercise routine for everyone, no matter how fit or unfit you are.

Physical exercise is any bodily activity that improves or maintains wellness, physical health and fitness. The NHS website states, 'If exercise were a pill, it would be the most cost-effective drug ever invented'. We must not underestimate the importance of the role of exercise in maintaining good health and, conversely, we must appreciate the importance of the role that lack of exercise plays in the causation of deterioration of health and premature ageing.

The opposite of an active lifestyle is a sedentary lifestyle, which can lead to a number of health issues that may shorten life expectancy. The NHS website states that exercise is the 'miracle cure we've all been waiting for'. It can reduce your risk of major illnesses such as heart disease, stroke, high blood pressure, type 2 diabetes and cancer by up to 50 per cent and lowers your risk of early death by up to 30 per cent. There is also good evidence that physical activity can boost self-esteem, mood, sleep quality and energy, as well as reducing the risk of stress, depression, dementia and Alzheimer's disease.

Medical evidence has shown that people who do regular physical activity have a lower risk of the following:

- coronary heart disease and stroke by up to 35 per cent
- type 2 diabetes by up to 50 per cent
- colon cancer by up to 50 per cent
- breast cancer by up to 20 per cent
- early death by up to 30 per cent
- osteoarthritis by up to 83 per cent
- hip fracture by up to 68 per cent
- falls by up to 30 per cent
- depression by up to 30 per cent
- dementia by up to 30 per cent

With all of this evidence available, then why don't we all do exercise? I believe it's because of the following reasons:

- We don't know what to do
- We don't have the time, we're too busy
- There is so much confusing advice about exercise out there
- There is a fear of failure
- There is a fear of not doing it correctly
- There is a fear of injury or causing harm
- We have tried it before and failed
- How do we know we're doing enough?
- Most exercise programmes focus on achieving what appears to be an impossible outcome and body shape
- There is poor motivation because of depression

The modern lifestyle has changed our perception of relaxation and pleasure being gained from sedentary activities, rather than active ones. This has led to sedentary behaviours, which include:

- watching TV, using the computer and playing electronic games instead of enjoying a physical activity and hobbies
- communicating on mobile phones or via email instead of physically meeting up with friends and family
- using cars for even short journeys instead of walking

- taking the elevator or escalators instead of the stairs
- our ways of working have also become more sedentary, where they used to be more manual, because of technology

Even if you do achieve your daily target of physical activity, your risk of disease can still be high if the rest of your time is spent sitting or lying down. The key to a healthier lifestyle is achieving your physical activity goals and then being mobile in between.

Different age groups require different types of exercise.

EARLY CHILDHOOD (UNDER FIVE YEARS OLD)

- Babies are continuously active throughout the day, moving around, reaching out, pulling their legs up, raising their heads and trying to sit up, turn around and crawl.
- Toddlers should be physically active for at least three hours a day indoors and outside. Try to minimise pram time, and encourage them to walk, run and play.
- Children under the age of five should not be inactive for long periods, especially in front of the TV, travelling by car, bus or train, or being strapped to a buggy.

- All children should be encouraged to play and do sports for their physical and social development.

YOUNG PEOPLE (FIVE TO EIGHTEEN YEARS OF AGE)

- This group requires at least sixty minutes of moderate to vigorous activity per day.
- Three days per week these activities should involve exercises for strong muscles and bones, such as push-ups, running and jumping. In today's society we are seeing too many of our young people sitting with electronic devices, watching TV, travelling by car or public transport instead of walking, running, cycling, playing and doing physical activities.

ADULTS (NINETEEN TO SIXTY-FOUR YEARS OLD)

- This group requires at least 150 minutes of moderate physical activity per week, such as cycling, brisk walking or swimming.
- Strength exercises on at least two days a week that work all the major muscle groups, including legs, hips, back, abdomen, chest, shoulders and arms.

or

- Seventy-five minutes of vigorous aerobic

activity, such as running or a game of singles tennis, squash or football.

and

- Strength exercises on at least two days a week that work all the major muscle groups as above.

or

- A mixture of moderate and vigorous aerobic activity. Two thirty-minute runs plus thirty minutes of brisk walking equate to 150 minutes of moderate aerobic activity.

and

- Strength exercises on at least two days per week as above.

OLDER ADULTS (SIXTY-FIVE AND OVER)

- At least 150 minutes of moderate aerobic activity.

and

- Strength exercises on at least two days per week as above.

or

- Seventy-five minutes of vigorous aerobic activity as above.

and

- Strength exercises on at least two days per week as above.

or

- A mixture of moderate and vigorous aerobic activity as above, and strength exercises on at least two days per week, as above.

Core and muscular weakness increases the risk of falls for older adults, with an increased risk of hip fracture and an inability to get up. Most older adult deaths are associated with falls at home, with inability to get up, and these people can be on the floor all night, which can lead to hypothermia and cardiac arrest. Immobility from a fracture also increases the risk of chest infections.

How to know what is enough exercise

For exercise to be beneficial, there should be a change in your heart rate and breathing, and you should also feel warmer. For example:

- Moderate aerobic activity is at an intensity where you can still talk, but can't sing the words of a song.
- Vigorous aerobic activity is at an intensity where you can no longer hold a conversation and can only say a few words without pausing for breath.

Getting started

It doesn't matter where you are in your lifestyle, you just need to have a desire to improve your physical and psychological health, and reduce your risk of disease and early death. Every journey starts with one step. If you do not exercise, or haven't exercised for some time, here is some advice:

- Start small
- Make one change at a time
- Plan your mornings
- Overcome your fear of exercise by knowing the facts and how it can help you achieve your goals
- Have a long-term vision and goal
- Accept that you will make mistakes and miss days
- It takes thirty days to replace one habit with another so most people will give up in the third week
- Be patient: it takes about three months to see a real difference
- Be aware of 'Metabolic Adaptation' (where your body adapts to your exercise and you stop losing weight – this doesn't affect the health benefits) and be prepared to change your exercise every three months if weight loss is your goal. It is important to look beyond weight loss for health

benefits. Your body will adjust over twelve to eighteen months.

The purpose of this chapter is to help you understand the importance of exercise, and to show that it is not difficult to change your lifestyle for a healthier outcome. I have talked about specific exercises that have been shown to reverse ageing in earlier chapters, and on our website you can see exactly how they should be done on our video tutorials, which include complete programmes. Visit www.drkhansturnbacktime.co.uk, where you'll find these and expert guidance from personal trainers Lucas and Despina on our Beginner, Intermediate, Advanced and Postnatal programmes.

BEGINNER

So, you're probably someone who has perhaps never given exercise a second thought. Or maybe someone too scared or intimidated to step foot in a gym. Or maybe you're someone who thinks you could never do the things that you see on TV or social media. That's fine because this programme is designed for you to do even from the comfort of your own home. You don't need anything specific, just your everyday chair, a mat and a couple of filled 1.5–2l water bottles. This phase is designed to help you feel comfortable about training;

to help you strengthen and mobilise your body before stepping it up to the next stage. The goal here is to help your body move better, to make everyday things a little easier for you to achieve.

INTERMEDIATE PROGRAMME

After a beginner programme more based on mobility and stretching you should be able to go to the next phase, which is more resistance training. This phase is called an accumulation phase and is there to build up your muscular endurance by slowly and progressively increasing your total volume and frequency of training over the weeks. It's a full body workout that will be very flexible to fit in with your diary and won't take long to perform (about thirty minutes).

The goal is also to build up the reps rather than the difficulty of the exercise (which is the goal of the advanced programme once you're ready). That phase should take you about four to six weeks before going on to the next one. Remember, don't increase your volume too drastically – you've got plenty of time!

ADVANCED

All right, now you are strong and ready enough it's time to move on to the advanced programme. This time we are switching the type of exercise as well as the structure of it. Here, the exercises that will be performed are harder and more intense as you will use more plyometric movements (jumping) and also put more of your body weight on each rep by changing the angles of movement so therefore more resistance. For that reason, you might not be able to perform as many reps compared to the advanced module but then again you will build it up week after week.

We are also going to do more than two exercises in a row to build up your stamina and increase the intensity. So, to be short, it's circuit training that involves a lot of full- and half-body exercises (which therefore require you to use a lot of different muscle groups at the same time), intense and with minimum rest periods. This will be hard and you will probably insult me during the session, which is fine because you will see the benefits of it later. Enjoy!

POSTNATAL

After having a baby, it's not uncommon for you to feel like your body is not your own. It's not how it once was: it has gone from pre-pregnancy to creating life and now the aftermath, but you can't stop. The pressures of being a mum can be overwhelming, but making sure your body is strong enough to cope with everyday life is essential. Now, before you think about going into any exercise programme after pregnancy, you must first consult with your doctor to get the all-clear!

I want you to think of this phase as not something you are doing to just 'lose the baby fat', but to help strengthen what has now become weak and strained due to pregnancy. Once we have the foundations in place and your body is ready, you can then move on to the next stage. The hormone relaxin will stay within your body for up to five or six months (depending on the person) after giving birth. This is the hormone that relaxes the joints within the body to help you give birth in the first place. Due to this we must be very careful and the correct form is of absolute importance! Lots of static core exercises and pelvic floor exercises to strengthen the transverse abdominals are key. Remember, this phase is to help you lay down the foundations to get your body back on track after the strains of pregnancy. Slow and steady wins the race!

There is also a section on our website on how to train at home once you feel ready to progress to the next level of exercise. This progression is not for everyone, so please do what feels comfortable for you. Here are a few examples of the exercises included:

WARM UP

Cat Camel Stretch – Gentle exercise that stretches and strengthens the muscles that surround and stabilise the spine. Starting position is on the floor on your hands and knees. Alternate between arching and rounding the back to make sure all three sections (cervical, thoracic and lumbar) extend and flex together. Perform this movement slowly while breathing; do not force the movement.

Thread the Needle – Rotational exercise to help strengthen and increase mobility within your spine. Can be performed either on hands and knees, or progress to hands and toes. Placing one arm through the gap of the other arm to then bring it back up, rotate spine and bring hand up to ceiling.

Four-Point Superman – Working on balance and co-ordination. A great core exercise to engage the glute muscles (bum) and lower back. Start on your hands and knees. Raise one arm and the opposite leg at the same time as high as you can. Be sure to clench the glute muscles and abdominal muscles to maintain good balance and posture. Lower them back down and repeat on the other side.

Single Leg, Leg Raises – Targeting to strengthen abdominals and mobilise hip flexors and hamstrings. Perform lying flat on the floor, one knee to be flexed with foot flat on floor. The other leg lies flat, ready to be raised as high as you can. Feel the stretch in the back of the leg (hamstrings) and slowly lower back down to the floor.

BEGINNERS

Chair Squat – A good way to start to learn the movement pattern of an actual squat, working mainly the muscles within your legs (hamstrings, quadriceps and glutes). The chair brings an element of safety to the exercise so you do not fall over. Start with your feet slightly wider than hip-width apart, with your toes pointing slightly outwards (this should prevent the knees from caving inwards). Now engage your abdominals, look straight ahead throughout the movement, inhale, push your hips back and bend your knees to lower into a squat until you are touching the chair. Keep your body weight on your heels; when you are ready to exhale, push through your heels and come back up to starting position.

Glute Bridges – A simple yet effective exercise to help activate and strengthen the glute muscles. It teaches you how to extend your hips, while keeping a neutral spine and braced core. To perform, start by lying with your back against the floor (neutral spine), knees bent and feet hip-width apart, flat on the floor. Drive your feet through the floor and push through your heels. Now extend your hips upwards, keeping your core braced, and squeeze your glutes in the top position. Your body should be straight from your knees to your shoulders. Come back down in a controlled motion and repeat.

Dead Bugs – An excellent exercise to strengthen your core area without putting strain on your lower back. This is also a great way to work on your co-ordination skills, working brain and core at the same time. Start by lying flat on the floor and point your arms to the ceiling. Bring your legs up and bend your knees so they are at a ninety-degree angle; make sure that your back is as flat as possible to the floor. Slowly lower one arm and the opposite leg to the floor at the same time. Using your core muscles, bring them back up to the starting position and repeat on the other side.

Floor Press – An upper-body exercise that strengthens the chest, shoulders and arms. The use of the floor eliminates the risk of potential strain on the shoulder joint. Grab two dumbbells (or water bottles) and lie flat on your back, knees bent and feet flat on the floor. Have your elbows bent at a ninety-degree angle with the backs of your arms (triceps) resting on the floor, dumbbells above your chest. While exhaling and bracing your core, press the dumbbells upwards. Pause and squeeze for a second and then in a controlled movement bring them back down to the starting position.

Floor Alternating Row – Work on strengthening the back muscles and gaining better posture. Start on your knees and hands to the floor with dumbbells (or water bottles) in each hand. Keep your spine in a neutral position, gaze fixed to the floor. Drawing one arm back, keeping your elbow close to your waist, squeezing your back as you row upwards. Keep your core braced so your hips do not tilt. Use a controlled movement to lower the arm back down, then repeat on the other side.

Shoulder and Spine Rotations – Help give more mobility to the shoulder, scapula and thoracic (middle) section of the spine. Start by lying on your side on the floor. Position yourself with your top leg bent at a ninety-degree angle and resting on top of a foam roller (or cushion) to keep your pelvis neutral. Your bottom arm lies flat on the floor out in front of you, with the other arm resting on top. Start rotating the top arm above your head, aiming to keep your hand on the floor. Once you hit a point where it becomes difficult, hold it there until you feel you can carry on with the rotation.

Once you get to your limit, take a deep breath and slowly bring the arm around to the starting position.

INTERMEDIATE

Goblet Squat – Progressing from the chair squat (see page 94), strengthening not only primarily the leg muscles, but also the back lat muscles too. Stand with your feet slightly wider than hip-width position, with your toes slightly pointing outwards and holding a light weight (kettlebell or dumbbell) close to your chest. Squat down, keeping your chest up, back tight and core braced until you are in a comfortable position, preferably with your thighs parallel to the floor. Exhale, push through your heels and come back up to the starting position.

Hip Thrust off Bench – Excellent for improving hip extension and glute strength. The stronger your glute muscles, the less strain you will have on your lower back, overall reducing the risk of injury. Start by sitting on the floor, with your back against the edge of a bench, step or sofa (if at home), feet hip-width apart and flat on the floor. Push through your heels and extend your hips upwards until your body resembles a flat table-top. Keep your chin neutral, squeeze your glutes and exhale. Hold for at least a couple of seconds and then slowly lower yourself back down to the starting position.

Leg Raises – Targeting the core and leg muscles, the main muscle groups involved include the abdominals, hip flexors, back muscles and thigh muscles. Start by lying flat on the floor and place your hands underneath your glutes – this will prevent strain on your lower back due to raising the glutes slightly. Now brace your core and raise your legs up, keeping them straight with a slightly softened knee. Exhale as you bring your legs up, then lower in a controlled manner.

Press-up on Knees – One of the most basic and effective upper-body exercises you can do, strengthening your chest, shoulders and triceps, as well as your core. Start on your knees and the palms of your hands with your body at a slant. Keep your core engaged and don't let your hips sink. Slowly bend your elbows and lower your chest towards the floor. Now press upwards, back towrds the starting position.

Banded Seated Row – Works on strengthening the upper back muscles. Sit on the floor with your legs straight out in front of you, toes pointing up. Loop the band on your feet, with an end in each hand, arms extended in front. Keeping your core braced, exhale and pull your elbows in as you pull the band towards you, squeezing your shoulder blades together. Pause and squeeze for a second, then in a controlled manner, return to the starting position.

Banded Shoulder Press – Helps strengthen the shoulders and increases overall stability in the whole body. Standing upright, your feet will be on one side of the band, holding it to the floor. Your feet will also be just wider than hip-width apart. Holding the other side of the band in your hands, bend your elbows so your hands will be either side of your shoulders. Now brace your core and squeeze your glutes to prevent your lower back from straining. Exhale and press your hands above your head. Control the movement back down, keeping everything tight and squeezed.

ADVANCED

Burpees – An intense exercise targeting the whole body, improving muscular endurance and helping to reduce body fat. Start by standing up straight. Drop into a squat, placing your hands on the ground in front of your feet. Kick your feet back behind you so you are now in a full plank position. Jump back to where your hands are and then jump vertically up in the air with your arms above your head.

Press-ups – Progressing from your knees to your feet, the full press-up is an effective upper-body exercise you can do to strengthen your chest, shoulders and triceps, as well as your core. Start as though you are moving into a full plank position on the palms of your hands. Keep your core engaged and don't let your hips sink. Slowly bend your elbows and lower your chest towards the floor. Then press upwards to starting position.

Single-leg Glute Bridges – A simple but powerful exercise to strengthen the glutes. Doing single leg helps you to define whether there is an imbalance between the two legs, helping the weaker leg get stronger without the stronger side compensating. Start by lying on your back with one leg raised in the air. Extend your hips off the ground as high as you can. Keep your core braced and squeeze your glutes as hard as you can. Now slowly lower yourself back down to starting position.

TRX Row – Mainly working your back muscles and lats, this also improves your hand grip, shoulders and core muscles. First, make sure the TRX is attached to somewhere safe and that it's safe and you have enough room to perform the exercise. Grab the handles in each hand and make sure you are facing the piece of equipment. Place your feet together and gently lean back in a diagonal position. Keep your core and glutes tightened so there is no strain on your lower back. Now pull yourself up by drawing your elbows back, keeping them close to your waist. Squeeze your back muscles, holding for a second, and then slowly lower yourself back down to the starting position.

Banded Upright Row – Creates tone and definition within the shoulders and neck if done correctly. To start, stand with your feet shoulder-width apart and have one side of the band underneath your feet. Hold the other side of the band in your hands a few inches apart. Keeping core braced and glutes tight, raise your upper arm out to the side, allowing your elbow to bend upwards until your hands are near your collarbone. Hold and squeeze for a second and then lower back down in a controlled manner to the starting position.

Lunges – A great exercise to strengthen the leg muscles, including quadriceps, glutes and hamstrings. Can be done either with your bodyweight, or with added weight (dumbbells or barbell). If done incorrectly, you can put strain on your joints so keep your upper body straight, with your shoulders relaxed and chin in a neutral position. Always keep your core braced and engaged. Step one foot out in front, flat on the floor, keeping your back foot up on your toes. Keeping your arms by your side, lower your hips by bending your knees until they are at a ninety-degree angle – be careful that your back knee doesn't smack the floor. Exhale and push through your front foot heel and rise back into the starting position.

Ab Toes Touches – An excellent exercise to help strengthen the abdominal area. More advanced than your normal leg raises as this incorporates your upper body as well as your lower body. Start by lying flat on the floor with your arms straight above your head. Make sure your core is braced; exhale and raise both legs and torso at the same time until your feet and hands meet, creating a V shape. Keep your abs engaged and try to control the movement back down to the starting position.

POSTNATAL

Pelvic Tilt Glute Bridges – Adding a posterior tilt into your glute bridge really helps to strengthen the intra-abdominal muscles (transverse abdominals). This is important after the strain of giving birth. Start in a normal glute bridge position, with your back to the floor, knees bent and feet flat against the floor. Tuck your hips (pelvis) so they are closer to the floor – this is called a posterior tilt. You then want to push your weight through your heels and extend your hips up and squeeze your glutes. Hold for a second or two and then slowly come back down.

Heel Taps – Focusing on the lower and intra-abdominal muscles again to help strengthen them after the strain of pregnancy. Lie flat on your back with your posterior tilt on your pelvis again (see Pelvic Tilt Glute Bridges, page 102). Now lift your legs in the air with a ninety-degree bend at the knee. You then want to lower one leg, keeping the bend in the knee, until the heel of your foot touches the floor. Keeping your core braced, exhale and then bring that leg back up. Alternate with the other leg.

Chair Squat – A good way to start to learn the movement pattern of an actual squat, working mainly the muscles within your legs (hamstrings, quadriceps and glutes). The chair brings an element of safety to the exercise so you do not fall over to begin with. Start with your feet slightly wider than hip-width apart, with your toes pointing slightly outwards (this should prevent the knees from caving inwards). Engage your abdominals, look straight ahead throughout the movement, inhale, push your hips back and bend your knees to lower into a squat until you are touching the chair. Keep your body weight on your heels and when ready exhale, push through your heels and come back up to starting position.

TRX Row – Working mainly the back muscles and lats, this also improves hand grip, shoulders and core muscles. First, make sure the TRX is attached to somewhere safe and it's safe to perform the exercise (see page 100). Now grab the handles in each hand and make sure you are facing the piece of equipment. Place your feet together and gently lean back in a diagonal position, keeping your core and glutes squeezed so there is no strain on your lower back. Pull yourself up by drawing your elbows back, keeping them close to your waist. Squeeze your back muscles, holding for a second, and then slowly lower yourself back down to the starting position.

Side Planks – This exercise will train the core muscles isometrically targeting the obliques. Strengthening these muscles plays an important role in strengthening your core in general as they support the abdominal wall. Start by lying on your side with your knees bent at a ninety-degree angle. Place your forearm on the floor with your elbow directly under your shoulder. Now brace your core so you feel like your belly button has gone to your spine. Lift your hips from the floor and hold for up to twenty seconds. Remember to breathe throughout the exercise; do not hold your breath. Lower your back down and repeat on the other side.

Band Windmills – This helps to open the chest and shoulders, while also rotating, strengthening and mobilising the scapular (shoulders). Holding a long band with each side in each hand, stand up straight, core braced and glutes tight. Now lift your arms in a rotational movement, keeping them as straight as possible throughout the sequence until you reach your sticking point. Once there, hold for a second or two to feel the stretch and then slowly come back around, keeping the arms still straight.

Side Leg Raises – The Side Leg Raise primarily works the abductor muscle group. These muscles are extremely important for daily activities and strengthening the abductors can make your movements more effective. The Side Leg Raise is also an effective exercise for toning the hip area. Start by lying on your side with your legs straight on top of each other. Cradle your head in your arm for comfort, with your other arm supporting you on the floor. Now lift your upper leg as high as you can, keeping your core braced, and squeeze your glutes. Lower back down to the starting position.

Pelvic Tilts – This exercise helps strengthen the abdominal muscles and stretches out the lower back. Start by lying with your back on the floor in a neutral position, legs bent and feet flat on the floor. Pull your belly button in towards your spine, pushing your pelvis up (see Pelvic Tilt Glute Bridges, page 102). Now tighten your gluteus and hip muscles as you tilt your pelvis forward. Hold for a second or two, and then return to the starting position.

CHAPTER 7

IT'S ALL IN YOUR DNA AND HABITS

We hear a lot about health and the treatment of illness. I have had the privilege of being trained in and practicing in one of the best health services in the world. Medical research and development, and proof in the form of clinical and medical evidence continue to form the basis of safe and effective medical practice. Good-quality research has fallen to organisations outside the NHS, but continues to be regulated at the highest level by ethical committees.

As a population, and individually, we enjoy a better state of health than ever before. We continue to gain a better understanding of what causes health problems and better ways of treating them. There is a limit, however, to what our health services can provide; as the population increases, our ability to treat diseases improves and expectations increase, and the NHS is becoming overworked and overstretched. One of the larger expenses is the 'drugs bill'. Pharma companies have to invest millions and years of research before a drug or medicine can be released. They must then recoup their investment, and make some profit, in the first five years in which they have an exclusive licence to supply that drug before it becomes generic, and other companies can also manufacture it, and the price therefore drops. If Pharma companies were not able to make a profit and reinvest into research and development, however, we would not be in a position where we could have such a good health service.

With stretched resources and limited numbers of practitioners, we find that the health service is fully occupied with the treatment of illness and conditions once they have occurred and there is little time or resource left to deal with the prevention side of things. To me it seems that the health service has become a 'Disease Management Service'. The problem with this approach, as I see it, is that it becomes a reactive service and can only address existing conditions and is less aware of emerging conditions, which are developing as a result of changes in lifestyle and habits. Fortunately, research into this has been conducted over years and we have a better understanding of what is causing health issues and how we may be able to treat and manage them.

The improvement in the health of the world has resulted in an increase in population, with the added burden of feeding, housing and transporting them. This has fuelled the food industry to produce processed foods, which instantly supply the need. Unfortunately, the research and development of such foods and their safety is not as rigorous as it is for the pharmaceutical industry, so we have had to see what effects they have on health over time.

Over the last decade we have seen a rise in what is being called 'holistic medicine'. Many who practice this have limited, if any, formal training in medicine and so can only give one part of the solution. This can bring its own dangers for those who have a medical condition that requires treatment with medication. I shall give you three examples to illustrate my point:

CASE STUDY: 1

In my NHS practice I had a patient who had type 2 diabetes, which was well controlled through diet, exercise and medications. He was enjoying a healthy lifestyle, punctuated with the irritation of having to take his medication, monitor his blood sugar levels and have regular reviews at my diabetes clinic. At the clinic he was fully supported by the team of doctors, nurses, nutritionist, dietician and podiatrist at my practice and the consultant-led diabetic clinic at the local teaching hospital. He went back to India for a holiday for three months and when he returned, he came in to see me. He had lost a lot of weight, developed painful ulcers on his feet and ankles, and couldn't feel his feet. On assessment I diagnosed diabetic neuropathy with diabetic ulcers. His blood sugars were very high and so I arranged for an emergency admission under the diabetic team. He was in hospital for six weeks, during which time he had a double-leg amputation and had to be nursed in ITU and then the high dependency unit because he was going into multiple organ failure because of uncontrolled diabetes.

Within six months he went from being a well-controlled diabetic leading a productive life with a good job to a double amputee who nearly died, without any work and a long path of rehabilitation ahead of him. He faced a life of disability and the inability to go back to his former job with the associated psychological consequences. So what happened to him?

While in India he met with a 'holistic medicine practitioner', who convinced him that he could cure his diabetes with diet, nutrition and herbal medicinal 'cures', and so he stopped his diabetic medication and monitoring.

CASE STUDY 2

A patient came to see me at my Harley Street clinic and during the process of going through her medical history she mentioned that she had been diagnosed with breast cancer. She had been seeing a 'natural medicine practitioner' in Harley Street, who had strongly advised her not to see a breast cancer specialist and instead to see her for a diet and nutritional programme to 'cure' the cancer. She was not even medically qualified. Thankfully, this patient did not take her advice and is now clear of cancer.

CASE STUDY 3

A friend of ours came in to see me and told me that she had been attending a 'natural medicine' clinic, where she was encouraged to have a thermography imaging of her breasts, which showed a vascular hot spot in one of them. This raised the suspicion of early cancer. It was claimed that this test could pick up cancer before any of the traditional tests. This friend of mine was then encouraged to start a course of supplements to help 'cure' the cancer. I was shocked and horrified at the advice given as we know that the earlier we catch cancer, the better chance we have of a cure, if treated appropriately. There is a rapid access service provided by the NHS for this purpose. I naturally advised her to see her GP to engage with this service. On researching the evidence behind thermography I found that it is not an accurate test and that there is a significant amount of false negatives and false positives found. It should never be relied upon as a stand-alone diagnostic test and if there is any suspicion of cancer, it should be treated aggressively, without delay, in order to get the best outcome. As it happened there was nothing to worry about, but the psychological stress and anguish my friend had to go through, being told that she might have early breast cancer, and all the further tests that took some weeks, was totally unnecessary.

These three studies illustrate the current trend for over-reliance on 'natural medicine' approaches to medical conditions. My vision of a balanced approach to health is to have a balanced view when it comes to three aspects of health and wellness:

1. **Support** good cellular health. This is where good holistic and natural approach comes into its own, and what this book is partly about.

2. **Manage** and screen for any identified genetic risks to health, so that potential conditions can be avoided through specific lifestyle adjustments and be picked up early and treated before they become a significant risk to health.

3. **Treat**, and/or manage any medical condition medically or surgically in order to cure or minimise the effect of that condition physically and/or psychologically.

By having a balanced, combined approach, we can get the best out of our lives on this planet.

DNA PROFILING

We each have an individual genetic profile which determines all of our physical and nonphysical characteristics (such as intelligence and personality). Our genes also determine how we interact with our environments and what sensitivities we have, our hormonal profiles, how we exercise and recover, and how prone we are to certain injuries.

Our genetic makeup can also predispose us to certain illnesses or diseases, such as heart disease, certain cancers, presenile dementias, diabetes and so on. If we know what these potential risks are, we can control our environment to reduce the likelihood of developing them. We can also create a bespoke screening programme for individuals to look for these conditions at an early stage, when more can be done for them.

With DNA profiling, we can also look at our telomere length so we can get a good idea of our biological ageing.

There has been so much study of genetic profiling that there are DNA tests that can determine a child's inborn genetic talent in order to determine which future career would be best suited for them.

There are many test kits available online. To get the most useful information from your DNA test, you will need to consult with a medical practitioner who can put things into perspective and put together a plan of action for you.

So what can we look for in DNA testing?

- our ancestry
- genetic predisposition for disease conditions that we may develop; carrier status conditions, that we can pass on to our children; drug response genes to medications; wellness traits, such as muscle performance, lactose intolerance and metabolism of caffeine and alcohol sensitivity; traits such as baldness, facial features and hair colour and addictions
- telomere tests (see above)
- vitamin D deficiency test
- health and wellness DNA tests to look at:
- exercise recovery
- muscle strength
- power and performance

- endurance
- joint health
- metabolism
- food sensitivities and food breakdown
- hunger and weight
- vitamin deficiencies
- addictive behaviours to certain foods

We can also look specifically at DNA fitness profiles, nutritional needs profiles, sexual behaviour tests, and sexual health tests. These tests require a sample of cellular material from which the various tests can be carried out. This includes blood, hair and buccal mucosal cells (taken from the mouth as swabs). Once we know what our genetic blueprint is, with the help of a professional we can develop a bespoke lifestyle around our specific needs. We can also devise a specific screening programme to look out for those predisposed conditions.

So what can we do with this information?

DNA cannot be changed, but it can tell us the valuable story of you, what you can eat, what exercise you need and what illnesses or conditions you are genetically prone to. This story can help us to help you with ageing, and although it is great to look good, we are not only talking about aesthetic ageing, we are talking about how you feel, reversing painful joints, arthritis, memory loss, preventing cancer and neurological illnesses. Biological ageing is where it all begins. How amazing that with information on your genetic makeup you can help 'turn back time' and make a full body reboot.

Where do habits fit in?

If we acknowledge that 20 per cent of how you age is due to genetics, the other 80 per cent is down to habits and lifestyle. This may appear easy: you change your lifestyle and habits and this in turn changes the way you age and has a dramatic impact on your health. But is it as simple as that? No, the general formula of healthy eating and a healthy lifestyle does not work for everyone, as I for one know. By having the right genetic information we can give a specific lifestyle and diet for you. This genetic information comes from your DNA, your specific unique genetic blueprint. How many times do you hear people say, 'I've tried so hard to lose weight. I've followed this diet, that diet and still not lost weight'. That's because it's not a one-fits-all solution – your diet and exercise programme is all about you.

The background to understand this lifestyle programme comes from the fact that 'Life has four major phases from beginning to end'. When we are born our growth and development is determined by hormones, which are, in part also determined by our sex.

PHASE 1 – FROM BIRTH TO AGE ELEVEN

During the first five years of our lives the process that started in the womb continues and so our organ development, such as completion of the myelination (the maturation of nerves, where a fatty sheath insulates them) of the nerves in our brains, the completion of our sensory organs, our livers, spleens and kidneys, which can be considered to be immature until the age of about five, continues. The brain and skull continue to grow and develop until we are about eight years old. Our bodies do grow to a degree, but most of the development is in the completion of the cellular and functional organisation of our organs.

This maturation is driven by hormones, but steered by our genetics. The basic blueprint is being laid down. From this perspective diet, nutrition, sensory input, educational input and the environment all have a part to play in the basic blueprint. For example, the type of diet we follow can determine the type of basic muscle fibres that we develop, e.g. fast or slow-twitch fibres, over and above the genetic blueprint. Interestingly, research has shown that the number of fat cells that we have in adult life, and so our capacity to store fat is determined by the types of food and the calorific intake during this stage of life. This means that diet and nutrition is very important even in early life.

Environmental and educational factors (such as

learned behaviours and how we are taught to learn) can have a huge impact on our health in later life. It was thought that conditions such as heart disease, diabetes, inflammatory conditions, dementia and other age-related conditions were genetically inherited. However, there is increasing evidence to show that these conditions have a major environmental and behavioural basis to them. This is great news as it means that we can change things to prevent, and even reverse, these conditions.

PHASE 2 – FROM AGE ELEVEN TO TWENTY-TWO

This is where we see sexual development and the majority of the physical growth and maturation of the body, which is mainly driven by the blueprint laid down in Phase 1. During this phase the neural pathways are being laid down in the brain, which determine our basic responses and how we process things. In this phase teenagers appear to become mentally and socially dissociated, and 'difficult to communicate with'. Thankfully, this is only transient!

The growth is driven by growth hormone and sex hormones, particularly the androgenic hormones (male dominant, opposite to oestrogenic, or female dominant hormones; these hormones are responsible for development and growth of the body during adolescence). This explains why many teenagers are prone to acne. The high levels of these hormones stimulate the young and still somewhat immature cells to replicate and mature. They create an environment that is conducive to replication and procreation.

PHASE 3 – FROM AGES TWENTY-TWO TO THIRTY-FIVE

This is the stabilisation phase during which further muscular growth and development can occur. However, growth hormones are produced at the cellular level on demand when stimulated by exercise. During this phase the pituitary production of growth hormone bottoms out and is taken over by a complex of other hormones produced on demand, stimulated by exercise and dietary components. For example, eating grass-fed red meat will stimulate growth hormones at a cellular level, which is great if you are exercising as it puts on muscle. However, if you are not exercising then it will stimulate fat storage! If you are unwell or have precancerous cells they can also be stimulated by the growth hormones; they accelerate ageing and disease processes too. Therefore, it's important to cut down on red meat consumption after the age of fifty.

Once Phase 1 is over, these hormones start to diminish

and other hormones take over the control of metabolism, growth and regeneration, such as the thyroid hormones, insulin and the sex hormones. The adrenocortical hormones are involved with the stress response. Other hormones produced by the hypothalamus in the brain, such as leptin (see also page 34), are involved with the metabolic fine tuning of the body. There are lots of hormones that are produced at the cellular level and in the gut (by the gut bacteria) that interact to create a healthy balance for a healthy body.

Environmental, dietary and nutritional factors start to have more of an impact on hormonal balance and cellular health. During this phase the cells, their mitochondria (these are the power plants found in all cells, where energy for life is produced. When they stop working, the cells die) and the genes are still quite healthy and protected. However, free radical damage can start to change the genes, opening us up to the increased risk of cancer.

As I've said before, I see the age of thirty-five as the 'Tipping Point' at which our cells change from growing to ageing. Beyond this point growth hormones serve to accelerate the ageing process and can stimulate any immature cells (which may be pre-cancerous or cancer cells) to multiply and develop.

PHASE 4 – THIRTY-FIVE ONWARDS

This is the ageing phase; each cellular turnover brings us closer to our demise. It can be monitored by looking at telomeres, which are like the caps at the end of laces, for our DNA. They get shorter as cells turn over, until they can no longer hold the DNA together and the cellular line subsequently dies. Environmental factors can accelerate this process and our health is mainly determined by these factors during Phase 4 as cells reach the end of their replication lives and we start to lose cellular volume. This can lead to osteoporosis (loss of cellular content/thinning of bone), dermatoporosis (loss of cellular content/thinning of skin), myoporosis (loss of cellular content/wasting of muscles), cerebroporosis (loss of cellular content/shrinkage of the brain) and so on for all of the tissues of the body. Happily, this loss of tissue can be slowed down, stopped and even reversed in some areas through understanding your cellular requirements and adjusting the environment accordingly. A more bespoke approach can be made by profiling an individual's DNA and then creating a bespoke lifestyle programme for them.

From this information we know that the greatest impact of lifestyle and habits is after the age of thirty-five: by implementing good lifestyle before we can reach thirty-five in a much healthier and stronger state. But don't despair: if you are reading this after the age of thirty-five, it can be redressed by changes in nutrition, exercise and supplements.

How to age smart

Getting older... It happens to us all yet those two words still strike fear into the hearts of most men and women, conjuring up images of grey hair, belly fat, wrinkles and sagging skin. Then there's everything else that goes hand in hand with advancing years – the decline of our physical health and mental abilities, the lack of confidence and the thought that life has written us off or simply passed us by. But it doesn't have to be that way. As actress Helen Mirren said in a recent interview: 'This word "anti-aging" – we know we're getting older. You just want to look and feel as great as you can on a daily basis."'

So how do we do this? By tackling ageing from the inside out. And, in the world of health and beauty, it is this science that is fast becoming the next big trend. Called 'Cellular Healing', it is all about using the body's own integral healing system and your own DNA blueprint to retune the cells of your body so you can lead a healthier life for much longer.

Feeling young is more important than looking it (though the two usually go hand in hand) and while medicine still cannot stop the toll that time exacts on our bodies there is much we can do to lessen the impact of getting older. We can soften wrinkles, rejuvenate skin and conceal the signs of ageing, but ultimately it is also important how you feel on the inside. What's the point of looking ten years younger if you don't feel it or act it?

Having a healthy lifestyle and a 'clean' diet is always a wise first step, however. Knowing exactly what your body requires gives you the best chance of significantly improving your health, longevity and staying younger and healthier for longer. We can do this by carrying out a range of tests to find out your individual health profile and how you're ageing. Steps can then be taken to address problem areas, including lifestyle choices through to gut health, diet, nutrition and exercise, which influence how you age and your health outcomes. We're one of the first clinics to introduce this exciting new programme and believe it's the future of anti-ageing. Below we tell you more about what's involved plus some simple lifestyle tips you can follow now.

So who is Cellular Healing aimed at?

Everyone can benefit. In the past scientists believed that the body was just one big biological clock that was wound up at birth, kept ticking, never missing a beat until our thirties and then over the next forty-six years started winding down, with all the signs of ageing accelerating with each decade. Today, experts believe that our biological clocks can keep on ticking for as long as 110 years using strategies to keep them in good repair.

What happens when our Cellular Healing system starts to wind down?

The ageing process doesn't only affect our external appearance but also our internal health, and so we become at risk of age-related health issues, such as tiredness, fatigue, weight gain, joint, tendon and muscular stiffness and pains; also high blood pressure, diabetes, heart disease, deterioration of vision, poor sleep, forgetfulness and poor memory, low moods, depression and dementia. We are also at an increased risk of cancer, as our immune systems become less efficient.

But don't our genes influence ageing?

Genetics will determine our blueprint, and how our cells, organs and bodies will work. They also determine certain risk factors for our health. However, it is our DNA that forms the blueprint of what we are, how efficient our systems are, and what weaknesses we have, just as different cars have different attributes. Our lifestyle then determines how efficiently we function within the parameters of that blueprint. If we do not look after our bodies in the most efficient way possible, they will wear out, rust and break down, very much as a car would if it is not regularly serviced. Knowing our DNA blueprint can help us to have an intelligent approach to our lifestyle.

So how does Cellular Healing work?

First, samples are taken from a mouth swab, hair sample (this also gives us an idea of the toxin build up in our bodies) and saliva collection, which will give us your DNA blueprint. A blood test will also look at your current health and hormonal status, organ, immune and bone function; and your nutritional status. Your cellular age can then be compared to your chronological age. We also look at your telomeres – which reflect how our cells have aged – to see how long they are, as their length is related to the longevity of your cells. Once we have implemented a change, we can monitor telomere length to see an improvement. Your DNA blueprint will determine your metabolic type, which determines how your metabolism is working as well as what type of exercise and recovery is ideal for you. We also check your nutrition, how your body absorbs various nutrients, whether you have any food intolerances and extra nutritional supplements you may need. We are also becoming more aware that the bugs in our gut constantly signal our genes. New research shows how important the two kilos of microbes that reside in our gut are to our wellbeing so it also makes sense to take great care of our tiny friends in the gut. A simple stool test can tell us about how friends are doing, and whether there is an upset in the balance of good and bad microbes.

These tests will give us important information about how your body works and what changes we can make to improve your cellular health, reduce risk and prevent future problems. With this information we can have an intelligent approach to your health, exercise, diet and nutrition that is specific to you. Unless there are specific disease conditions, or syndromes related to your DNA and genetics, your environment has a much greater impact on ageing and health in later life. Even with pre-existing genetic conditions, we can improve the health and outlook by having an intelligent approach to cellular health. Rather than screening everyone of a certain age for everything, we can be more targeted. Just as different cars have different requirements for fuel, oil maintenance and servicing, so do we when it comes to our nutritional, exercise and lifestyle requirements. We believe that it takes six to eighteen months to turn your health around.

(For more details about Cellular Healing, telephone 0207 436 4441 – DNA tests cost from £500.)

TIPS

Be age-smart now

- **Look after your bones**
  Half of all women and one in five men aged over fifty will break a bone because of a weakened skeleton (osteoporosis). A vitamin D supplement helps promote calcium absorption and bone health. Weight-bearing exercises, such as working out with lightweights, three times a week, can also help keep bones strong.

- **Deal with your stress**
  Stress contributes to every disease, directly or indirectly. It shrinks the brain and increases the waistline. So deal with it – somehow. Make time for mindfulness, or even better, meditation and even a few minutes of relaxed deep breathing several times a day will help. With your eyes closed, focus your mind on one object, breathe in deeply over five seconds and then blow away any stresses of the day over five seconds. Wait for a count of five and then repeat. Do this for five minutes and then follow with a glass of water.

- **Build exercise into your everyday life**
  Regular exercise helps prevent the arterial ageing

that contributes to memory loss, improves muscle mass and makes you look and feel better. Even thirty to forty-five minutes a day of brisk walking has been shown to grow new brain cells as well as reduce the risk of heart disease, cancer, diabetes and depression.

- **Be sun-wise**
  Forget wrinkle cream – the only skincare product that can truly slow ageing and prevent skin cancer – is sunscreen. Always use a broad spectrum cream with a minimum SPF 20 and apply every day, rain or shine, and SPF 50 on holiday.

- **Get more beauty sleep**
  Sleep deprivation can cause weight gain, weakens the immune system and may accelerate ageing. You need two and a half hours before sleep becomes restorative, which then activates the release of GH (growth hormones). Aim for seven hours every night. If you have difficulty sleeping, try eating five almonds and two dates within thirty minutes of getting up in the morning as this can improve your sleep pattern at night. Also, avoid caffeine after 5pm and moderate your alcohol consumption during week nights.

- **Know your body**
  After the age of fifty you should know your key health statistics, including weight, blood pressure, cholesterol and hormone levels. Hormones are chemical messengers that are critical for making healthy cells. Our peak hormone levels occur during our teens and early twenties and tend to level off around the age of twenty-five to our mid-thirties when they begin to drop.

- **Have regular check-ups**
  Visit your dentist for a check-up at least twice a year to avoid gum disease – people with gum disease are twice as likely to have heart disease. So what's the connection? There are a few theories, including that inflammation of the gums can cause the arteries to accumulate plaque. Have regular eye checks too as these can also pick up early health warnings. Have a check-up as often as your GP will do it for you and check for your genetic risks every six to twelve months by engaging with a screening program. The NHS doesn't offer this type of screening yet, so it would have to be on a private medical basis.

- **Eat well**
  Diet has a profound influence on how well we age.

A balanced diet with fewer refined carbohydrates (anything with sugar and/or white flour) but plenty of fruit, vegetables, nuts, white meats and fish and smaller quantities of red meat can give you a headstart in staving off weight gain and associated health problems. Smaller quantities of high-quality protein are always the best way to go. Remember that weight gain is a symptom of something going wrong, so we can screen against it and make changes early to control it. Obesity is when it has become a disease, and gone beyond prevention, and treatment may be the only option.

- **Be happy**
  A positive attitude can boost feel-good hormones so laugh more, socialise with friends and enjoy life. Research shows that a good laugh can help manage stress and prevent the release of damaging hormones in the body.

- **Stimulate your brain**
  The brain also needs exercising to avoid becoming sluggish so learn a new language, read and learn to play a new instrument or do a daily crossword puzzle. These last two will help slow the development of dementia and depression.

CHAPTER 8

MODERN LIFESTYLE AND HABITS

We have already discussed how lifestyle and habits impact on your health. As I've said before, your outcomes are 80 per cent determined by non-genetic factors and 20 per cent by genetic factors. It then goes without saying, the better the lifestyle and habits, the better the outcome. The benefits of exercise have been known since ancient Greek times, and I have already discussed the importance of this in Chapter 6.

In the last 50 years we have seen a number of changes in lifestyle and habits that impact on health. Our lives have become busier and more stressful. Keeping up with technological advances has resulted in a significant change in the way we work and spend our leisure time. It also has had an impact on how and what we eat, and the kind of exercise we do. There have been changes in our education system too, with a shift of focus away from sports and exercise and more emphasis on exam outcomes and rankings on league tables. In this chapter, I would like to highlight lifestyles and habits which will result in a change in your health, wellbeing and life expectancy.

Work/life balance

We have discussed work/life balance and recreation in previous chapters. The modern lifestyle has put a great deal of pressure on the way we work. In the good old days people used to clock on and clock off. Work was work, and home life was home time, with enough time to pursue leisure activities and hobbies. Families used to sit together at mealtimes, and communication was more face-to-face. Children used to play outside with friends, and adults would have more of an active social scene.

Technology has resulted in a shrinking workforce and increasing output, which means more responsibility, more stress, and less personal, family and social time. We are also at the end of smartphones, receiving texts, emails and calls relating to work twenty-four hours a day, seven days a week, even when we are on holiday. This intrusion of work into our personal life has resulted in a more stressful environment. The environment in the cities, where many of us live, is becoming more polluted and the quality of food and drink we are ingesting is deteriorating. Where it was easy to get involved in leisure activities in the past, we now have to plan and prioritise them carefully, and sometimes it is easier not to do them at all. This can result in chronic stress and depression. It can also lead to behaviours and habits aimed at reducing stress, anxiety, poor sleep and depression. These may include emotional eating and snacking on convenience foods, smoking, drinking alcohol, taking drugs, prescribed and recreational, escaping into electronic games, or the television. All this can lead to social isolation and the breakdown of relationships.

With anxiety and depression there is a loss of efficiency at work, which leads to even more stress and the feelings of inadequacy and isolation. The thought of exercise and physical activity can itself cause more anxiety and is avoided. So to keep things simple in this chapter I am going to discuss the key areas where we can all make significant changes.

Smoking

We are all aware of the health risks of smoking. It is one of the biggest causes of illness and death in the world. In the UK, it is responsible for around 100,000 deaths, with many more living with diseases caused by it. Smoking is known to cause 90 per cent of lung cancers, but is also a potent carcinogen in the formation of cancers elsewhere in the body, such as the following:

- mouth
- lips
- throat
- larynx
- oesophagus
- bladder
- kidneys
- liver
- stomach
- pancreas

Smoking also damages the cardiovascular system, increasing the risk of developing the following:

- coronary heart disease
- heart attack
- stroke
- peripheral vascular disease
- cerebrovascular disease
- cerebrovascular dementia
- impotency in men
- reduced fertility in men and women

Smoking also damages your lungs, leading to:

- chronic obstructive pulmonary disease (COPD), including bronchitis and emphysema
- pneumonia
- worsening of other lung conditions, such as asthma, flu and the common cold

Smoking during pregnancy increases health and complication risks of:

- miscarriage
- early labour and premature birth
- low birthweight babies
- stillbirth

The health risks of passive smoking are also well documented. Passive, or second-hand smoking comes from the tip of a lit cigarette and/or the smoke the smoker has breathed out. A passive smoker's cancer risk will go up by 25 per cent. Babies and children are particularly susceptible to the effects of second-hand smoke, increasing the risks of:

- chest infections
- meningitis
- persistent cough

- worsening of symptoms of asthma
- increase in risk of death from severe acute asthma
- glue ear
- cot death
- increase in the incidence of cancer, both in childhood and in adult life
- diminished IQ, from the lead exposure from cigarette smoke and ash.

My advice is obvious: STOP SMOKING! I do, however, appreciate that this kind of advice is neither useful, nor effective, if we do not offer support and help for people who genuinely want to stop because they would have done so if they could. Fortunately, there are smoking cessation clinic services available on the NHS, so if you want to stop smoking and improve your health outlook, you can find such a clinic near to where you live or work by visiting www.nhs.uk (search for 'smoking cessation clinic'). If you live outside the UK, you will be able to find support by searching the internet.

Alcohol

We hear a lot about alcohol and its dangers in the news and from the medical profession. Alcohol is a double-edged sword in that consumed in regular moderate amounts (of about 1.5 units per day) it has a health benefit effect.

What you drink can also enhance that beneficial effect. Some drinks, such as wines, grappa, brandy and whisky, are high in antioxidants, while others can be toxic, like absinthe (which can contain a toxic chemical called thujone from wormwood) and tequila (some of which can contain methanol). Some of the beneficial effects of smaller amounts of alcohol include:

- Anxiolytic (anti-anxiety) effect – it helps people to relax in social environments.
- Vasodilatation – it dilates blood vessels, and improves blood supply to the body's tissues and organs, including the brain, keeping you sharp and protecting you from dementia.
- A small pre-meal aperitif can act as a digestive and helps prepare the stomach and intestine to better digest food. It can also increase insulin sensitivity. There has been shown to be a decrease in the risk of type 2 diabetes and weight gain in those who drink in moderation.
- It has been shown to increase good cholesterol (HDL-cholesterol) levels by up to 20 per cent when accompanied by a healthy diet (similar benefit is seen by taking statins (drugs used to lower cholesterol) or running a half-marathon, though

exercise has other benefits over and above this). It also helps to reduce the formation of clots, and so reduces the risk of heart attacks and strokes.

Evidence does not distinguish types of drink when it comes to health benefits. However, different forms of alcohol have different components, which have their own effect on health, such as antioxidant content, or sugar content.

The downside of alcohol is associated with (a) some toxins in particular types of alcohol, and (b) toxic alcohols (such as methanol, ethylene glycol (found in antifreeze), and isopropyl alcohol content. The alcohol content of alcoholic beverages should be ethanol and ethyl alcohol. Most commonly, the downside is associated with overconsumption of alcohol, which can reach toxic levels. Alcohol is detoxified mainly by the liver and high levels increase the production of detoxification enzymes, and over a longer period, can cause damage to the liver cells.

The over-consumption of alcohol can increase your risk of:

- Liver disease, including alcohol-induced hepatitis, cirrhosis and liver cancer
- High blood pressure due to its effects on the kidneys, with subsequent renal failure

- Heart failure, cardiomyopathy and heart attack
- Brain damage due to depletion of vitamin B1 (thiamine – Wernicke's encephalopathy), dementia and stroke
- Foetal alcohol syndrome in pregnancy
- Other cancers, such as mouth, throat, larynx, oesophagus, colon, rectum and breast, as well as liver
- Psychological and other psychiatric problems and addiction
- Severe acute alcohol poisoning with acute swelling of the brain and eventual death
- Violence, injury and death related to drunkenness
- Metabolic changes, with raised cortisol, insulin resistance, muscle wasting, osteoporosis, obesity (this is also partly due to the calorific value of alcohol and the liver inhibition of its ability to mobilise medium chain-free fatty acids), and type 2 diabetes
- Alcohol can also interact with certain medicines, either directly, or through liver enzyme induction.

My advice on alcohol is to control your consumption within healthy parameters (1–1.5 units a day) as part of a healthy diet and lifestyle. There is evidence to support that it is best taken with food.

If you feel that you are consuming too much alcohol

and can't reduce it by yourself, help is available through your GP and the various agencies, such as Drinkline, Alcoholics Anonymous, Al-Anon Family Groups (help and support for families and friends of people with drink problems), Addaction, Adfam, the National Association for Children of Alcoholics (Nacoa), and SMART Recovery.

A healthy diet

This can be easier said than done in our hectic lifestyle. It is easy to pick up convenience foods, which are usually processed, full of sugar, salt, additives, colourants and preservatives. In previous chapters we have covered the nutrient content of certain foods and how to ensure high quality. In this chapter I am going to cover the principles of achieving a healthy diet in our modern lifestyle. Here are the principles of a healthy diet.

- Make sure that you eat a variety of foods. Nature provides us with the right nutrients, at the right time and in the right combinations so that we can be assured of getting the best combination of synergistic nutrients and other essential ingredients such as signalling peptides and enzymes, which ensure optimal absorption and use of the nutrients by our cells. Our research into what nutrients do what is important in our understanding of how they impact on health, and the importance of a variety in our diet. There has, I feel, been a jumping on the bandwagon by companies who then use this research to market supplements. The evidence for supplements over natural foods is lacking and there is growing evidence that the best way to take nutrients is how nature presents them in seasonal, organic foods, with the appropriate enzymes and signalling through sight, smell, taste and chewing that prepares your intestinal tract to absorb the nutrients.

- When shopping for food make sure that you recognise the food for what it is supposed to be. In other words, chicken should be recognisable, either as whole or as portions, not in a reconstituted piece. The same applies to fruit and vegetables. I call this shopping for 'single-ingredient foods' – you can mix them yourself later when cooking.

- When shopping for foods ensure that they are organic and seasonal. Fruit and vegetables that look good and wholesome *are* just that. Those that smell good are letting you know that they are ripe and full of nutrients that are ready for you to eat and absorb. Those that taste good are signalling your systems to get ready to absorb and take full advantage of the nutritional value that they offer. Foods that don't smell of what they should are probably lacking the nutritional content and taste required for you to benefit from them.

- Supplements do not interact with our senses or physiology in the same way as fresh food and so our systems are not prepared or ready to receive or utilise them. If you are taking supplements it is best to have them with appropriate foods that contain that, or those nutrients.

- Avoid shopping when you are hungry.

- Choose meat from healthy animals (see page 77). By that I mean organic, grass-fed beef and lamb and free range poultry. The fish we buy should be from deep sea sources. Inland farmed fish can be contaminated with pesticides, herbicides and other chemicals used in farming. Coastal fish can be contaminated with heavy metal pollutants and human consumed drugs and medicines, pumped out in sewage waste. Tiny plastic beads are also being consumed by fish living in coastal areas. As we age, we need less animal protein (meat), so we do not have to spend as much on meat or fish as we need smaller portions.

- When preparing and cooking foods, try not to overcook them as this can destroy nutrients. With meats, avoid too much charring as this can increase the amount of free radicals you ingest. Eating raw fruit and vegetables is good and remember to aim to eat a 'rainbow' of colour with your fruit and vegetables. The wider the variety of food, the better the variety of nutrients.

- Remember, your stomach's capacity is the same size as your fist and we have already discussed the effects of overstretching the stomach and its effects on ghrelin production and the loss of the satiation response (see also page 27). For main meals aim to have a portion the same size as your fist on your plate. A portion of protein is the size of your palm, or 75–150g. It is recommended that you aim to consume two portions of protein a day (more if you are participating in regular sports). You can eat as much low-GI fruit and vegetables as you want, ensuring a variety and plenty of fibre in your diet.

- Fats should be limited to two tablespoons a day of healthy unrefined fats and organic cold-pressed oils. Limit, or preferably cut out, your intake of refined sugars and high-GI carbohydrate foods. Also, try not to drink too much water with your food as it may dilute the enzymes and reduce their effectiveness.

How and when to have food and drink

Remember, 5 per cent dehydration means 20 per cent reduction in efficiency, and we don't feel thirsty until we are 15 per cent dehydrated. It is therefore important not to become dehydrated. I recommend that you aim to drink a glass of water every hour. Metabolic stability is achieved by a steady state of energy release and this can be achieved by how we eat. Eating first thing in the morning helps us to fire up the engines of the cells to start burning calories that fuel our activities. What we eat is also important as it will determine whether we burn fat or store it so a sensible breakfast would include proteins, fats and low GI carbs. I like to start the day with two dates and five unsalted almonds within thirty minutes of getting up in the morning. A recent study from Leeds University showed that this actually stabilises metabolism and balances hormones for a healthier lifestyle and better sleep. It also sees me through to lunchtime without feeling hungry. On the mornings you exercise, you could eat the dates and almonds after you have exercised.

At weekends you can enjoy a hearty fry-up if you wish two hours later (but not every day). At lunchtimes I would recommend half a portion of protein, some healthy fats and as much low-GI carbohydrates in the form of vegetables and/or fruit as you wish. You can have the other half-portion of protein two to three hours later, then between 6 and 8pm have one portion of protein, some fats and as much low-GI carbohydrates as you wish, with 1–1.5 units of alcohol, if you wish – as long as you're not driving afterwards. If you feel peckish at bedtime, have either lean protein in the form of chicken or turkey breast, or low-GI foods like nuts or cherries, when in season.

Caffeine in tea and coffee has been shown to be good for health in moderation of two to three cups per day. However, excess caffeine can contribute to an increase in blood pressure. I would also advise that you do not have caffeine after 6pm as it can disturb a good night's sleep.

On the subject of oils a good tip is that different oils have different smoking point temperatures. It is important not to heat them to smoking point as this is the point at which free radicals are created and repeated use of the oil can increase health risk, including that of gastro-oesophageal cancer. I would avoid trans fats and hydrogenated oils. These are used in processed foods, including a lot of the 'health foods' like protein bars, etc. Trans fats are also used for cooking fast food – for example, French fries – and are created when oil is repeatedly heated. They increase the risk of heart disease by raising the bad and lowering the good cholesterol;

they can also directly interact with arterial plaques, changing them from stable to unstable plaques, which can then result in heart attacks.

The consumption of cholesterol is not related to raised cholesterol in most people. It can pose a risk in those who are genetically predisposed to high cholesterol. Cholesterol problems are more related to poor metabolism, so can be addressed with lifestyle changes. By following the advice given in this book you can improve things. Remember: Moderate alcohol, healthy diet, exercise

Salt high in sodium should be avoided. I would advise that salts high in potassium, and other minerals such as magnesium, should be used in preference (like sea salt, or Himalayan salt). Remember:

- Sodium increases blood pressure
- Potassium decreases blood pressure
- Magnesium reduces blood pressure and heart disease and improves sports performance. It helps regulate metabolism and diabetes, improves sleep and reduces depression. Magnesium is absorbed through the skin so foot soaks and soaking in a bath of Epsom salts regularly helps. It is also found in spring water, dairy products, vegetables, wholegrains, fruit and nuts.

Manganese is another important mineral that is not very much talked about. It has an important role in supporting bone health, enzyme function, protection against free radical damage, supports brain function, respiratory and metabolic systems, and may help with weight loss; it also reduces inflammation of joints and PMS symptoms, helps balance iron levels and prevents anaemia. It has been shown to have an important role in maintaining fertility and speeding up the healing of wounds.

Manganese is found in wholegrains, brown rice, chickpeas, nuts and beans.

Calcium and vitamin D are important for maintaining health as we age. We may not be able to get enough of these through our diet, and may also have issues absorbing them as we get older, so this is one of the few exceptions where I would recommend supplementation. I would advise that you have a blood test first and then have your doctor prescribe the right amount for you and monitor your levels. However, in general, I would advise that you choose healthy, seasonal organic food over supplements every time.

The most important message I want to convey here is that most diets are boring, unsustainable and not necessarily good for you. Any weight loss is then replaced by the equivalent or even greater weight gain. This yo-yo weight loss and weight gain isn't just not good for your physical health, but can have serious consequences on your psychological and mental health too. My aim is to help you to understand how you can improve your health, lose weight and enjoy your food all at the same time and avoid the soul-destroying yo-yo weight changes and associated physical and psychological consequences.

Be wary of fruit juices

I have already discussed the importance of eating whole fruit and vegetables, so if you are going to enjoy a liquid version, be sure to blend or liquidise the whole fruit and vegetable, then consume it as soon as possible, because the enzymes have been released and the process of breakdown and oxidation has started. Chilling and freezing slows this degradation down. Juicing, on the other hand, removes much of the beneficial part of the fruit and vegetables and essentially presents you with a flavoured and coloured liquid packed with sugar.

When you read the labels of fruit juice, they may state that the carton or bottle contains the juice of ten fruits. It is easy to consume a litre of juice quickly, but almost certainly you would not be able to consume ten fruits as easily. In effect you are consuming flavoured liquid calories with little other nutrition and the enzymes required to absorb them properly.

Physical activity

We should all have a good idea of how important physical exercise is. The key to losing excess weight is to understand the simple law of physics, that 'energy consumed – energy expended = net energy retained'. If the net energy retained is a positive figure, then we will gain weight. However, if the net energy retained is negative, we will lose weight. By applying this principle, we can see how, by slightly reducing caloric intake and slightly increasing our exertion, we can start to tip the balance from weight gain to weight loss. I would advise that if you take baby steps, then you can achieve anything and still enjoy your lifestyle.

The following activities will improve your health:

- walking, cycling or running instead of using the car all the time
- taking the stairs instead of the elevator or escalators

When shopping for fresh food it may be useful to shop two to three times a week to ensure freshness, this could also mean two to three visits to the shops a week, including carrying the shopping home.

If you're busy at work and have a desk job, don't keep a large bottle of water by your desk. Instead get up and walk to the water dispenser every hour to get some water. At lunchtime take a walk to stretch your legs.

If you are more motivated, and enjoy exercise then you could incorporate a session of 'burst' exercises for ten minutes every morning, and possibly two to three sessions of HIIT exercises for twenty to forty minutes each week (see also page 25).

Remember, metabolic adaptation occurs after about two to three months so it is important to keep changing the type of exercise that you do, if you want to continue to lose weight. However, the health benefits do not reduce with metabolic adaptation, so carry on exercising.

Other ways to improve circulation include hydrotherapy, with hot and cold showering, and body brushing or massage. The way to do hydrotherapy is to have a shower or bath and then at the end heat up the water so you are starting to sweat, being careful not to burn yourself, for two minutes. This is followed by cooling the water to the point of it being cool enough for you to stop sweating and just before it is too cold to be uncomfortable, again for two minutes. Done daily, this is good for detoxifying the body as toxins are stored in the subcutaneous fat in our bodies and by increasing the blood flow they can be flushed away and excreted with sweat. However, be careful not to plunge into iced water (at a sauna, for example) if you are not used to it as this can cause cardiac dysrhythmias and even cardiac arrest. Body brushing and lymphatic massage improves lymphatic flow, which also has a similar effect on toxin build-up. It is always important to remember that if you have a medical condition, or are pregnant, that you take medical advice from your GP before engaging with any lifestyle program.

Psychological wellbeing

We are not just physical beings, we are psycho-physical beings. In other words, our physical and psychological healths are interlinked and one affects the other. It is just as important to look after our mental and psychological health as our physical health. We have already discussed that by having a balanced nutrition and exercising we can control our hormonal balances, which in turn help with psychological wellbeing. However, there are other ways of dealing with stress, anxiety and depression. We can also influence and prevent and even reverse dementia by carrying out the following practices:

- Make time for regular meditation and mindfulness. This is where you take five to ten minutes to clear your mind of all thoughts and just concentrate on your breathing. Place one hand on the centre of your chest and the other on your stomach and feel them rock up and down like a seesaw with each breath. In your mind's eye, imagine being by the sea and watching the tide come in and go out with each breath.

- There is good evidence to show that by stimulating the brain by learning a new skill we can preserve the brain and even reverse the effects of dementia and depression. The more diverse the stimulation the better – in other words, learning a new language is great, but involves fewer sensory inputs than, say, learning to play a musical instrument, or learning to dance.

- Humans require human interaction, and isolation can lead to depression and the progression of dementia. We have become so busy in our lives that we forget that we share this world, our country, and even our street with other people. When I was in practice in the NHS I would see people with depression who had become isolated and were showing signs of areas of the brain shutting down. I encouraged some of them to identify an elderly neighbour who was isolated and bake a cake or biscuits for them, take them over and have tea with them. The feedback and results were amazing. Those who followed my advice developed a friendship and started to care for the elderly person. Soon their depression lifted and they became sharper in their thoughts. The elderly person also benefited from an improvement in their mental state and any signs of dementia also improved. They felt less isolated and both of their self-esteems improved.

- General movement and physical activity improves the blood flow to all of your organs, including the brain. So, if you are in a sedentary job, remember to get up and walk around your desk every hour, or go get a glass of water. Aim to increase your daily exercise by walking more, using the stairs or going for a walk at lunchtime.
- Hobbies that tax us, both physically and mentally, are important and if they require social interaction, so much the better.

Forming good habits

Research is showing that habits are more important than we previously thought. We used to think that medical diseases and conditions were 80 per cent determined by genetics and only 20 per cent by habits and lifestyle. Research over the past 70 years has revealed that the opposite is actually true. We inherit our genetic makeup, but we also acquire our habits from our early environment and if these habits caused our parents to have a medical condition, the chances are that we will also develop them.

So, what is a habit? A habit is a learned behaviour that is repeated so many times and for so long that it becomes a subconscious programme that runs even without us knowing it. Some habits have been repeated for so long over generations that they have almost become a tradition. Habits occupy time and space, so it is almost impossible to break or lose a habit as it would leave a vacuum or void, something our brains cannot accept. We must therefore replace one habit with another, more desirable and beneficial one. Our minds will accept an exchange, however, because they are used to subconsciously following one path. We have to work consciously to create a new path while avoiding the old path so that our minds can then follow this new path subconsciously. It is like building and laying a new path in a different direction across a field and actively directing people to walk along it, while the old path falls into disuse and breaks down over time until it is indistinguishable from the field. Remember, it takes thirty days to create a habit, but you may have to work on it longer as it could take longer for the old habit to fade.

So how do we create new habits? There are a few simple scientific steps that I want to share with you:

- **Motivation**: I like to define this as your 'motive for action'. To be truly motivated to make a change in habits, it is important to know the facts about what habit you want to change and why, and the facts about what new habit you want to develop and why. Knowledge that you have faith and belief in is key to your motivation.

- **Have a goal**. This should be your big picture as to what you want to achieve. This goal should be intrinsic, not extrinsic (as a response to punishment or reward).

- **Plan doable steps** that can be taken daily to help you to achieve your goal.

- **Write your to-do steps down**, be very specific and study them daily. Repeat them daily for at least thirty days. This creates what we call 'behaviour chains' that can be adhered to.

- **Keep your daily steps simple** – eliminating too many options makes it easy to stick to the tasks.

- **Visualise yourself doing the steps** needed to achieve your goal.

At the age of seventeen I became the national champion at the triple jump for my age and the year above. The previous year I had been placed eighth. I remember sitting with my coach and setting what seemed to be an impossible goal of winning as I would be competing across two year bands: my own and the one above. Once we set the goal, he helped me to plan the competitions that I would compete in and win and set new Personal Bests during my year's journey to the National Championships – we called these the stepping stones. We then planned the training, or the to-do list required to achieve these micro goals.

We also visualised each training session, each competition and each new PB I was going to achieve. Before each competition I visualised doing the winning jump and a new PB and receiving my medal. By the end of that year I had achieved fifteen consecutive PBs in the triple jump and won the National Championships. That was not all, though: I also achieved PBs in 100m and 200m sprints, 110m hurdles, long jump, high jump, discus and hammer throws. Following this I was awarded Athlete of the Year by my club for receiving the most points for the club in the inter-club season that year. I guess what I'm trying to say here is that by having a goal, setting plans, visualising and putting into action your to-do list you can not only achieve your goals, but may also enjoy other benefits that come with the changes you make.

Remember, new habits are very fragile to start off with. Like learning to walk, if you had given up after a few stumbles and falls then you would never have walked. If you find things aren't going as you would like, go back to basics and analyse what went wrong, then start again. Don't give up and eliminate doubt. My advice to you is not to 'try' things, but to decide to 'do' them, because when you 'try', failure is more acceptable – 'oh well, I tried'. Let me ask you to do a task to illustrate my point:

- First, find a pen
- Now place it on the table
- I want you to 'try' and pick up that pen

What you probably did was to pick up the pen. Do you see? You either 'do' or 'do not' pick up the pen, there is no such thing as 'try'. It is a weak excuse for failure, 'whether I do, or I don't, at least I tried'. Oh, and by the way, did I succeed at every event to achieve my goals? No, I didn't. There were times when I didn't achieve all my goals. Life got in the way. Things happened that prevented me from achieving my mini-goals. So did I stop and give up? No, I didn't, because failure doesn't mean and isn't spelt 'STOP'! It is an opportunity to reassess and examine your to-do steps, and reset them in a better way to help you achieve your goals.

When I was eighteen my headmaster asked to see me with my father. I remember it as clearly as if it were yesterday. He told my father, 'He is more than capable of becoming an Olympic athlete and he is more than capable of becoming a great doctor, but he will not achieve both to the same standard together.' On learning this I knew that I had a decision to make right there and then. I think I made the right decision. All of the training and preparation I had for my athletics I now applied to my career as a doctor. I tell you this because we have all achieved and succeeded in the lives we have chosen. The habits and principles that we have applied to help us to learn to walk, run, become good at sports, work or a hobby, we can apply to set new habits and achieve new goals, as long as we really want to achieve them. These habits can become second nature, just as walking has for most of us. The principles for success are the same, whatever you apply them to.

So, how do you stay on the wagon?

First, if you're asking this question, you may be seeing this as a chore, and not a choice. If you are doing something that you really want to do, rather than something someone else is telling you to do, then you are more likely to stick to it.

- Set a goal that is important to you. Do it for selfish reasons, and don't feel guilty about your reasons. Don't set goals to impress other people, they don't care. Share your goals with those who are close to you, who care about you, and who will be supportive.

- Plan your steps, and commit to start. Take small steps, they will still get you to your destination, but if you miss one it is of less significance, and easier to recommence, than if you're trying to take big steps.
- Be prepared for the discomfort of change. Expect it to be uncomfortable, and embrace it as part of achieving your goals. You will have times when things appear to be harder, and more of a struggle.
- Have faith in your choices, and back your actions up with knowledge, based on evidence. Don't be swept away by people, or groups with agendas that are not sincere, and don't get distracted, jumping from one idea to another in search for an easy rout – there isn't one.

In this book I have presented a plan, which hopefully gives you knowledge about why you should consider changing your lifestyle, and how to do it. The advice is consistent with a sustainable lifestyle, so there isn't really a waggon to fall off.

CHAPTER 9

SHOPPING LIST, RECIPES AND THE PLAN TO PUT IT ALL TOGETHER TO FIT YOUR LIFESTYLE

The basis of 'keeping on the wagon' with this change in lifestyle is having tasty food, and a variety of food, and for me the mainstay has been always having a thick, filling and delicious lentil soup on the stove or chilling in the fridge so that if you are starving when you get in, then it can be heated up quickly. Now, coming from a catering family (my parents and grandmother had restaurants and pubs), I was raised to cook and love food. I love to experiment with flavours and the one thing I'm known for is never serving the same dish twice because every time I make a dish I try adding a little something extra. The recipes below are just a starting point – also try personalising them for a nutritious and tasty meal.

I use a lot of red lentils – they are perfect for anytime meals or snacks, or whenever you're in a hurry. They cook quickly so not only do I add them to lentil soups, dahl and pease pudding, I also use them to thicken most of my soups, stews, casseroles and curries rather than flour as they are so much better for you.

I'm often asked why lentils are so good for you and why they help with weight-loss. The humble lentil is a low-cost ingredient, also low in calories, high in nutrition and an almost fat-free powerhouse packed full of fibre, protein, minerals and vitamins. It can be used in so many different ways too and is perfect for vegetarians, vegans and meat eaters alike.

I like to add turmeric and ginger to my soups, stews and casseroles as these flavourings are anti-inflammatory. They help ease joint pains, arthritis and inflammation of the gut. I'm a big garlic user too as it is an antiseptic and helps fight off colds and flu.

YOUR SHOPPING LIST OF ESSENTIAL FOODS

Almonds (unsalted)
Apples
Artichokes
Asparagus
Aubergines

Avocados

Baking powder

Bananas

Basil

Beans (tinned, but not the 'Baked Beans in tomato sauce'): black, chickpeas, lentils, Pinto

Beetroot

Bok choy (also known as pak choi – Chinese cabbage)

Bread – rye, and whole seeded bread, without processed flour.

Broccoli

Butter – almond, cashew, coconut, Kerry Gold (or other butter from grass-fed cows), peanut, sunflower seed

Cabbage

Carrots

Cashews (unsalted)

Cauliflower

Celery

Cereals

Cheese

Chocolate – bars, chips (dairy-free)

Citrus (lemons, limes, oranges, pineapples)

Cocoa powder (natural)

Coconut milk (fresh or tinned)

Coriander (fresh)

Courgettes

Dates (Medjool are my favourite, but any dried ones will do)

Dried fruit – apricots, cranberries, dates, figs, prunes, raisins

Engevita yeast flakes (see also page 169)

Flour – buckwheat, chickpea, gluten-free or white wholewheat

French beans

Fridge – chicken breasts and legs, lamb neck fillets, lean bacon, chicken (organic, free-range), eggs (organic, free-range), grass-fed ground beef, ground turkey, orange juice, Pancetta, seafood, spread (dairy-free), tofu (organic), sustainably farmed in-season or wild fish

Garlic (fresh)

Ginger (fresh root, ground and powdered)

Grains – millet, oats (gluten-free), quinoa

Greens (lettuce, microgreens, spinach)

Herbs – basil, bay leaves, bouquet garni, chives, parsley, rosemary, thyme

Kale

Mayonnaise, from organic ingredients

Milk – almond, coconut, or organic grass fed milk

Mint jelly

Miso (Japanese seasoning)
Mushrooms (cremini, portobello, shiitake)
Mustard
Noodles and pasta – corn, durum, rice, soba
Nutritional yeast with B12
Nuts – almonds, cashews, hazelnuts, pecans, pine, walnuts
Oil – avocado, coconut, cold-pressed virgin olive oil, sesame seed
Olives – black, green
Onions – red, shallots, sweet, yellow
Parsnips
Peas (frozen)
Peppers (bell, chilli)
Polenta
Potatoes
Raw cacao powder
Rice – Arborio, brown, white, wild
Rosemary (fresh)
Sea salt
Seasonal fruit (apples, berries, mangoes, pears, stone fruit)
Seeds – chia, flax, pumpkin, sesame, sunflower
Fermented Soy sauce (non-GMO)
Spices – chilli powder (mild/hot), cinnamon, coriander (ground), cumin, ground black
pepper, oregano, paprika, turmeric

Spinach
Squash – butternut
Starch – corn (non-GMO), tapioca and/or potato
Stock (chicken, mushroom, you can get vegan stocks from most supermarkets)
Sugar – un-refined brown (very small amounts), honey, maple syrup or stevia
Sweet potatoes
Sweetener – agave nectar or local honey, maple syrup, molasses, or stevia
Tahini
Tinned fish – salmon, sardines, tuna, wild, Atlantic sourced
Tomatoes – fresh, ketchup, puree, sun-dried, tinned chopped tomatoes
Tortillas – corn, flour, gluten-free
Turnips
Vanilla essence
Vinegar – apple cider, balsamic, brown, unrefined basmati, or black rice

Hummus

Serves 6

475g can of black beans or chickpeas, drained

4 tablespoons tahini

2 tablespoons warm water

1½ tablespoons cold-pressed virgin olive oil

2 teaspoons lemon juice

2 teaspoons soy sauce (non-GMO, wheat free/gluten-free are available in supermarkets)

2-4 garlic cloves, minced

1 teaspoon cumin powder

2 tablespoons chopped flat-leaf parsley

Toasted rye bread or chopped raw vegetables, to serve

1. Place all the ingredients except the flat-leaf parsley in the bowl of a food blender and blend until smooth and creamy.
2. Transfer to a serving bowl and garnish with parsley.
3. Serve with toasted rye bread or chopped raw vegetables.

Healthy Delicious Frittata

Serves 4 hungry people or makes 6 snacks

Easy to make, nutritious and delicious – great for using up any leftover vegetables too.

1 tablespoon cold-pressed olive oil
2 tablespoons diced Pancetta (or bacon, if preferred)
1 small onion, peeled and finely chopped
2 garlic cloves, peeled and crushed
4 mushrooms, peeled and chopped
½ pepper, deseeded and diced
2 chopped tomatoes
diced courgette or any other leftover vegetables.
6 large free-range organic eggs, lightly beaten
1 tablespoon cheese
1 tablespoon flat-leaf parsley or basil, finely chopped, to garnish

1. Heat the olive oil in a large frying pan and fry the Pancetta or bacon, onion and garlic over a low heat until the onion and garlic are softened and golden.
2. Add your vegetables of choice and cook for a few minutes until the edges start to colour lightly.
3. Meanwhile, crack the eggs into a bowl, add a few twists of black pepper and whisk together well. Tip the beaten eggs onto the vegetables in the frying pan and stir to combine.

4. Preheat the grill to a medium heat. Reduce the heat to very low and cook until the edges of the frittata start to set.
5. Place the pan under the grill to finish cooking the top of the frittata. Once the top starts to bubble and brown, remove from under the grill. Sprinkle over the cheese. Return to the grill and cook for a few more minutes until brown.
6. Tip the frittata onto a large warmed plate, sprinkle with parsley or basil and slice into 4–6 wedges. Serve alone or with a tomato, avocado and onion salad.

Tasty Vegetable Patties – can be served alone as a snack or as part of a meal

Serves 4–6

Engevita yeast provides a rich source of B vitamins and minerals. Gluten-free, it is also suitable for vegans and available from health food stores.

175g gluten-free oats
250g turnip
250g beetroot
2 large carrots
4 tablespoons chopped fresh parsley
2 tablespoons chopped fresh chives
250g chopped kale

1 tablespoon turmeric
1 teaspoon crushed garlic
2 tablespoons Engevita yeast flakes with B12 (or any nutritional yeast)
1 teaspoon sea salt
½ teaspoon ground black pepper
1½ tablespoons sesame seed oil

1. In a bowl, blend the gluten-free oats into a fine flour.
2. Peel and shred the turnip, beetroot and carrots. Wrap a few handfuls at a time in kitchen paper and squeeze to remove as much excess moisture as possible.
3. Place the vegetables in a bowl, then add the chopped parsley, chives and kale. Mix together well.
4. Add the turmeric, garlic, yeast flakes, salt and pepper. Mix together well, then add the oat flour and stir in a little sesame seed (reserve the rest for frying). Shape the mixture into 8–10 small balls and flatten to make patties.
5. Add ½ tablespoon sesame seed oil to a large frying pan and heat to medium. Place the patties in the frying pan and fry on each side for about 4 minutes until golden brown.

Thick and Hearty Lentil Soup

Serves 6

1 teaspoon butter
2 large red onions, peeled and chopped
3 large carrots, peeled and chopped
3 sticks of celery
2 garlic cloves, peeled and crushed
1 teaspoon turmeric
4 tablespoons tinned chopped tomatoes
1cm fresh root ginger, peeled and finely chopped
400g red lentils
900ml vegetable stock made with organic stock cubes or bouillon
1 bouquet garni
Sea salt and freshly ground black pepper

1. Heat the butter in a large saucepan set over a low heat. Add the onions, carrots, celery and garlic, stirring with a wooden spoon to coat in butter. Sweat over a low heat for around 40 minutes. Don't rush this stage as this is what will give you the lovely taste.
2. Season with salt and pepper and turmeric. Pour in the chopped tomatoes, add the ginger and mix together well.
3. Add the lentils and stock.
4. Add the bouquet garni, bring to the boil, then reduce

the heat to low and simmer for 35 minutes, stirring occasionally, until lentils have softened.

Tip: If you like a smooth soup, use a hand-held blender and blend until smooth. I like my soups to be a bit chunky, so I only blend half the soup before serving or sometimes use a potato masher to leave some chunks.

Lentil and Spinach Soup

Serves 4

Quick and easy, delicious and vegan! Always have a pot of lentil soup ready for emergencies – that's when you are starving and need to feel full. Make a big batch on a Sunday and freeze it into plastic bags or pots. When you are freshly preparing food and freezing it, it will last for over a month (anything from 1 month to 1 year, depending on what it is). I usually advise that you prepare your food on a weekly basis, so it will be consumed within in the following week.

2 tablespoons col pressed extra virgin olive oil
2 onions, peeled and choppped
2 carrots, peeled and chopped
2 garlic cloves, peeled and crushed
2 tomatoes, deseeded and chopped
900ml vegetable stock

100g green or red lentils
1 bay leaf
200g fresh spinach leaves
½ teaspoon turmeric
Sea salt and freshly ground black pepper

1. Heat half the oil in a large pan. Add the onions, carrots and garlic. Reduce the heat and cook until the onions are turning opaque.
2. Add the tomatoes to the pan.
3. Stir in the stock and lentils and bring to the boil. Add the bay leaf and reduce the heat to low. Simmer for 25 minutes until the lentils have softened.
3. Meanwhile heat the remaining oil in a frying pan set over a low heat. Add the spinach and cook for 2 minutes or until wilted.
4. Stir the wilted spinach into the soup, check the seasoning and simmer for 5 minutes before serving.

Creamy Sweet Potato and Parsnip Mash

Serves 6 as a side dish.

This tasty mash goes especially well with meat or fish and a green vegetable.

1 bulb of fresh garlic
125ml cold-pressed extra virgin olive oil
2 large sweet potatoes, peeled and cut into 2.5cm cubes
3 large parsnips, peeled and cut into 2.5cm cubes
3 tablespoons chopped fresh parsley
Sea salt and freshly ground black pepper

1. Preheat the oven to 180°C/Gas 4.
2. Wrap the garlic bulb in foil and place on a small baking tray. Bake in the centre of the oven for 45 minutes by which time the garlic will have softened. Leave to cool, then slice and squeeze the soft garlic from its casing into the bowl of a blender.
3. In the blender combine the garlic with the olive oil
4. Steam the sweet potatoes and parsnips for around 15–20 minutes or until softened. Transfer to a large bowl and mash well.
5. When the vegetables are smooth and lump-free, stir in the garlic and olive oil mix a little at a time – you may not need it all (save it to use on any other vegetables). Stir in the parsley and season to taste.

Heartwarming Lamb Tagine

Serves 4–6

I cook this dish ahead of time, leave it in the fridge for a day or two and then reheat slowly for 40–60 minutes for an even better flavour. Serve on a bed of couscous or on its own.

2 lamb neck fillets, trimmed and cut into chunks
5 tablespoons cold-pressed olive oil
2 onions, peeled and chopped
4 garlic cloves, peeled and chopped
2 teaspoons ground cumin
2 teaspoons ground coriander
1 teaspoons chilli powder, hot or mild to your taste
1 teaspoon ground turmeric
1 teaspoon cinnamon
Juice of 1 lemon
250g pitted dates
200g dried apricots
Handful of fresh chopped coriander leaves, to garnish
Sea salt and freshly ground black pepper

1. Preheat the oven to 180°C/Gas 4.
2. Place the lamb in a plastic bag, add 1 tablespoon oil and seasoning to taste. Tie the bag tightly and shake well to season the lamb all over.
3. Heat a large frying pan, add the lamb and brown over

high heat for 1–2 minutes until lightly coloured. You may need to do this in two or three batches to ensure the chunks are sealed. Add a tablespoon more oil between each batch if needed and transfer to a large ovenproof casserole as each batch is browned.

4. Heat the remaining oil in the pan. Fry the onions and garlic over a low heat for 5 minutes or more until they are soft and lightly caramelised.
5. Add the cumin, coriander, chilli powder, turmeric, ground black pepper to taste and 1 teaspoon sea salt. Cook for 2 minutes, stirring continuously.
6. Place the lamb in the ovenproof casserole and add 1.5 litres of stock, then add the cinnamon and lemon juice. Bring to the boil, stirring. Reduce the heat to a simmer, cover with a lid and place in the centre of the oven to cook for 1 hour 15 minutes.
7. Remove the casserole from the oven. Stir in the dates and apricots, cover and return to the oven for another 30 minutes (sometimes it may take another 15–20 minutes for the lamb to be tender, so check after 30 minutes). Serve garnished with chopped coriander and couscous, if liked.

Rack of Lamb

Serves 2

Serve with this delicious selection of vegetables – bon appetit!

2 carrots, peeled
4 sprigs of rosemary
2 tablespoons olive oil
1 rack of lamb (6 chops)
1 large sweet potato, peeled and cut into wedges
2 handfuls of broccoli florets
1 onion, peeled and diced
125g frozen peas
1 organic stock cube
1 teaspoon mint jelly (optional)
Sea salt and freshly ground black pepper

1. Preheat the oven to 180°C/Gas 4. Meanwhile slice the carrots into matchsticks (julienne) and place in an ovenproof dish. Add 1 tablespoon of water and the rosemary and cover tightly with foil. Roast in the oven for 30 minutes with the lamb (see Step 2).
2. Pour 1 tablespoon olive oil into a deep roasting pan, place in the centre of the oven and heat until sizzling. Remove and carefully add the rack of lamb. Sear the lamb in the oil and then place fat side up. Roast for around 25–35 minutes depending on how well done you like your lamb.

3. Meanwhile steam the sweet potato wedges for around 8 minutes, then pop in a plastic bag with ½ tablespoon olive oil. Seal the bag and shake vigorously to coat the wedges in oil. Add to the roasting pan with the lamb.
4. Heat the remaining olive oil and fry the diced onion in a small saucepan until opaque. Add the frozen peas to a saucepan with a stock cube dissolved in 1 tablespoon water. Cover and cook over a very low heat for about 10 minutes.
5. Remove the lamb from the oven, check it is cooked to your liking, drain the juices into a saucepan and leave the meat to rest for 10 minutes. If you like mint, add a teaspoon of mint jelly to the meat juices and heat through. Slice the rack into chops and serve with the meat juices and vegetables.

Chicken and Butternut Squash

Serves 4

2 tablespoon olive oil

4 chicken legs, skin on

1 butternut squash, peeled and chopped into 1cm pieces

1 sweet potato, peeled and chopped into 1cm pieces

2 onions, peeled and chopped

6 garlic cloves, peeled and chopped

Cabbage or green peas, to serve

1. Preheat the oven to 190°C/Gas 5. Heat ½ tablespoon of oil in a roasting pan. Place the chicken legs skin-side down and sear in the oil. Set aside on a plate.
2. Add the remaining oil to a mixing bowl and toss the butternut squash, sweet potato, onions and garlic in it. Add to the roasting pan.
3. Arrange the chicken legs skin-side up on top of the vegetables and roast for 45–60 minutes. Check the chicken is fully cooked before serving.

Lovely Leftovers

After a roast chicken lunch, take the carcass and leftover chicken meat, wrap in muslin and place in a large pot with any leftover vegetables (I even add cauliflower cheese and any leftover gravy). Add a peeled chopped onion and carrot, 2 cloves chopped garlic and a teaspoon of turmeric and cover with water. Bring to the boil, then reduce the heat to low and cook for an hour. Remove the chicken carcass and allow to cool. Once cool, remove any chicken remnants, discard the bones and return the meat to the pot. Add 4 tablespoons lentils, bring back to the boil, then reduce the heat and simmer for 35 minutes. Taste and adjust the seasoning before serving, if necessary.

Mild Cauliflower and Lentil Curry

Serves 4

A tasty vegetarian curry, delicious served with wild broccoli rice. Broccoli rice has become very popular of late and can be purchased from most supermarkets ready prepared. However, if you like to make your own, see the Tip at the end of this recipe.

3 tablespoons vegetable oil
2 onions, peeled and chopped
2 garlic cloves, peeled and chopped
2.5cm fresh root ginger, peeled and chopped
2 teaspoons ground coriander
2 teaspoons ground cumin
1 teaspoon ground turmeric
100g red split lentils
150ml vegetable stock, made with an organic vegan stock cube
1 cauliflower
1 large carrot, peeled
400ml coconut milk, fresh or tinned
75g peas or French beans
Fresh coriander, chopped
Zest of 1/2 lemon and 1 tablespoon lemon juice
Sea salt and freshly ground black pepper
Broccoli Rice, to serve (optional, see Tip on page 181)

1. Heat 2 tablespoons of the oil in a large saucepan. Add the onions and fry until softened, stirring frequently so they do not burn.
2. Add the garlic and ginger to the pan with the ground coriander, cumin and turmeric and cook for 3 minutes, stirring all the time so as not to burn the spices.
3. Add the lentils, pour in the stock and bring to the boil, stirring. Reduce the heat to a simmer, cover and cook for 15 minutes.
4. Meanwhile trim the cauliflower into small florets and remove any thick hard stems. Slice the carrots into matchstick (julienne) strips.
5. Heat the remaining oil in a large frying pan and fry the cauliflower and carrots for around 3 minutes or until lightly golden. Add to the lentil stock. Stir in the coconut milk. Bring the pan back to a simmer and cook for 15–20 minutes by which time the vegetables will be tender.
6. Meanwhile make the Broccoli Rice (see Tip below). Stir in the peas or French beans into the curry and cook for 5 minutes.
7. Add the coriander and zest and lemon juice to the curry and season to taste. Serve on a bed of Broccoli Rice.

Tip: To make broccoli rice, put 4–6 broccoli stalks in the bowl of a food processor and pulse until finely diced, about the size of a grain of rice. (You could also use a cheese grater to grate the stalks if you don't have a food processor.) Add to a pan of hot water with a pinch of salt, bring to the boil and cook until tender, about 10 minutes.

Chocolate and Ginger Protein Balls

Makes 12, but I often double up to make enough for two people for a week.

Great for snacking, protein balls are rich in fibre, high in antioxidants, dairy-free and low in sugar. They are the easiest thing to prepare as they require zero cooking but are very tasty too. I make at least a couple of batches every Sunday and they will last for up to a week in the fridge. If you make big batches they keep very well in the freezer. Try making them in two or three different flavours.

50g oats
200g unsalted cashews or almonds
200g Medjool dates, pitted
2 teaspoons ground ginger
½ teaspoon grated fresh ginger
2 tablespoons raw cacao powder
A little coconut butter for rolling out

1. Place the oats and nuts in the bowl of a blender and blitz until a fine flour forms.
2. Add the dates and the ground and fresh ginger with half the raw cocao powder. Blend until a thick dough.
3. Tip the mixture out of the blender bowl onto a piece of greaseproof paper. Shape into a ball with your hands and then divide into 12 pieces.
4. Roll each piece lightly into a small ball, the size of a truffle – they are very filling. When rolling and shaping the mixture, keep a little coconut butter on the side and rub it into your hands: it stops the mixture sticking to you and the surface.
5. Arrange the balls on a plate and refrigerate for an hour. Remove from the fridge and dip each ball in the remaining raw cacao powder, then store in an airtight container in the fridge for up to one week.

Make ice cream, again dead easy but ready for when you need a sugar boost (see page 190).

Tasty Lemon Gluten- and Dairy-free French Toast

Serves 2

240ml almond milk

1 teaspoon vanilla essence

1 tablespoon yeast flakes

2 tablespoons ground chia seeds

1 teaspoon cinnamon

Pinch of sea salt

1 tablespoon agave syrup (also known as nectar)

Oil or coconut butter for frying

4 slices gluten-free bread

A sprinkling of sugar and lemon slices, to decorate

For the lemon sauce

2 tablespoons coconut butter

3 tablespoons agave syrup

Juice of ½ lemon

1. To make the batter, put the almond milk, vanilla essence, yeast flakes, chia seeds, cinnamon, sea salt, and agave syrup into a mixing bowl. Mix well, cover with a damp cloth and then let stand for 10 minutes.
2. Preheat a large frying pan to medium-high, add oil or coconut butter to the pan to prevent the bread from sticking. Do not let the oil or coconut butter heat to smoking point.

3. After the batter mix has been standing, dip each slice of bread in the mix, one by one, and place in the frying pan. Do not soak the bread too much or it will fall apart when frying. Fry the bread for 3–4 minutes on each side until a lovely golden brown colour.
4. While the bread is frying, make the lemon sauce. Mix the coconut butter, agave syrup and lemon juice in a small bowl, stirring together well until it is a thick creamy sauce.
5. Transfer the French toasts from the frying pan to serving plates and pour the creamy lemon sauce over the top of each one. Decorate with a sprinkling of sugar and lemon slices.

THE PLAN

Remember to have a glass (175mls – 250mls) of water every hour.
The evening meal can be accompanied with 1 – 1.5 units of alcohol of your choice.

Day One

6.30–6.45 am
Five unblanched almonds
Two dates, or four cherries, or ten grapes

BREAKFAST (7.30am) if you have exercised or are feeling hungry, if not this could be taken at 10-11am in place of your mid-morning snack
Black coffee
Two scrambled or poached eggs
Two slices of lightly smoked salmon

SNACK (10.30am, if required)
Handful of cherries/grapes/berries or/and nuts

LUNCH (12–1pm)
Roasted chicken-breast (half portion (2-3oz)
Avocado, Tomatoes, Salad greens; a small amount of

salad dressing can be used (2 tablespoons of olive oil with 1 teaspoon of balsamic vinegar with ground black pepper make this up at the beginning of the week and keep it in the fridge)

AFTERNOON TEA (4pm)
Tea/black coffee, hot lemon water or fruit tea of your choice
Small slice of polenta cake, a protein ball, or 6-8 nuts of your choice.

DINNER (6-8pm)
Grilled or poached fish, or meat of your choice, or vegan protein 1 portion (3-6 oz)
Mixed salad, with a small amount of dressing and/or roasted sweet potato, courgettes, onions, peppers

Day Two

6.30–6.45am
Five unblanched almonds
Two dates or four cherries, or ten grapes

BREAKFAST (7.30am, or 10 – 11am. As above)
Black coffee
Grilled tomatoes
Two slices of grilled unsmoked/ uncured bacon

SNACK (10.30am, if required)
Handful of cherries/grapes/berries or nuts

LUNCH (12–1pm)
Homemade lentil soup (see pages 171)

AFTERNOON TEA (4pm)
Tea or fruit tea of your choice
Protein balls (see page 182)

DINNER (6 – 8pm)
Grilled or roasted lamb (4-6oz), with gravy made from juices with onions, garlic, herbs, sea salt, pepper and chopped tomatoes, if desired.
Roasted sweet potato
French beans with garlic
Boiled kale and carrots

Pudding: Chia Seed and Mango Dessert – only if you want something sweet! Or seasonal fruit salad with a dressing made from orange juice, squeeze of half a lime, and honey to sweeten to taste.

Day Three

6.30–6.45am

Five unblanched almonds

Two dates

BREAKFAST (7.30am or 10 – 11am as above)

Black coffee

Fresh fruit platter – melon, orange, banana, cherries, apple and oatmeal porridge, or two boiled eggs with wholegrain bread soldiers.

SNACK (10.30am, if required)

Homemade protein balls (page 182), or a 6-8 nuts or fruit, such as berry fruits, an apple or an orange, or a green – yellow banana.

LUNCH (12–1pm)

Charcuterie platter (any cold meats 1-2oz) and 1-2oz cheese. Or dips (humus, tomato salsa, guacamole, cream cheese or aubergine with fingers of peppers, carrots and celery

Avocado and bean salad

Tomatoes and salad greens

Lemon water, tea/black coffee or fruit tea

AFTERNOON TEA (4pm)

Lemon water, tea/ black coffee or fruit tea of your choice

Small slice of cake

DINNER (6-8pm)

Grilled prawns (4-6oz) with chilli and lime

Mixed salad with nuts (I find walnuts with a pomegranate molasses and olive oil dressing particularly delicious)

Chocolate and Banana Quick Ice cream (3 frozen, over ripe bananas, three teaspoons of cocoa powder, a teaspoon of almond or hazelnut butter, and half a cup of almond milk, then blend in a powerful blender), if you fancy something sweet.

Gin and slimline tonic – single measure, then you can enjoy two! Keep topping up with tonic.

Day Four

6.30–6.45am

Five unblanched almonds

Two dates

BREAKFAST (7.30am or 10 -11am as above)

Two slices of thick ham

One poached egg

SNACK (10.30am, if required)
Homemade protein balls (page 182)

LUNCH (12–1pm)
Homemade vegetable soup
Water or tea of your choice

AFTERNOON TEA (4pm)
Hot lemon water, tea/black coffee or fruit tea of your choice
Small slice of polenta cake, a protein ball, or 6-8 nuts of your choice.

DINNER (6-8pm)
Grilled grass-fed rib-eye steak (4-6oz)
Mixed salad with a sprinkling of cheese (shaved parmesan)
Peach or piece of fruit as above
G&T with slimline tonic or water

Day Five

6.30–6.45am

Five unblanched almonds

Two dates

BREAKFAST (7.30am)

Slice of sourdough toast with mashed avocado

SNACK (10.30am, if required)

Handful of cherries/berries/grapes or nuts

LUNCH (12–1pm)

Naked quarter-pounder hamburger (no bread bun)

Slices of tomatoes and onions, ketchup and mustard

AFTERNOON TEA (4pm)

Hot lemon water, tea/coffee or fruit tea of your choice

Homemade protein balls (page 182)

DINNER (6-8pm)

Lentil Soup (page 171) followed by Stuffed Peppers

Day Six

6.30–6.45am

Five unblanched almonds

Two dates

BREAKFAST (7.30am or 10 - 11am as above)

Gluten-free muesli with almond or coconut milk

SNACK (10.30am, if required)

Protein balls (page 182)

LUNCH (12–1pm)

Crispy Romaine salad with anchovies or prawns

AFTERNOON TEA (4pm)

Tea or fruit tea of your choice

Handful of fruit and nuts

DINNER (6-8pm)

Grilled seabass

Mixed salad

G&T or vodka & tonic with slimline tonic

Day Seven

Take a break, eat sensibly, but enjoy the day and have a little of what you fancy!

CHAPTER 10

CAROLE MALONE'S TURN BACK TIME DIET

Depression. It's such a small word for such a gargantuan thing, such a life changer. Yet for most of my life it was a word that didn't touch me personally – it didn't enter my experience. Of course I'd read about it. I knew people (only vaguely) who suffered from it. But the truth was I didn't want to get close to it because I thought it was an excuse for not dealing with life, with problems. I'm ashamed to admit I thought people who were depressed were weak – people who couldn't or wouldn't cope. And by calling it 'depression' that was an excuse for them not doing what had to be done, i.e. pulling themselves together.

I believed the minute someone said they were depressed it was categorised as an illness and it stopped them from having to take responsibility for dealing with it. If you're ill it's not your fault, is it? Of course I look back now and know how terribly wrong I was, but for decades I was impatient with it. If I even got close to feeling 'depressed', i.e. 'fed up with the world', I'd give myself a good talking to. And I'd snap out of it. But then being fed up with the world isn't depression – it took me getting it myself to realise that.

I used to wonder what was wrong with all those other people who either couldn't be bothered or didn't have the will to do what I'd done – to snap out of my fed-up-ness and just get on. Little did I know they literally couldn't.

Let me take you back to years before I hit the wall – the big black wall that threatened to fall down on top of me and engulf me. In 2007 I landed a job as columnist and writer on the *News of the World.* It was the best job I'd ever had. I was working for the biggest Sunday newspaper in the world. Everyone read it – well, at least 7.5 million people every week did – even though many pretended they didn't. I used to watch people in paper shops buying so-called quality newspapers but whatever broadsheet they bought, they always slipped a *News of the World* inside it!

I was offered the job there by the editor, Colin Myler – an old friend and colleague who'd been working in New York for years and had come back to take the helm. But I was scared – I didn't know if I was up to it. I'd always known I was good at my job but this was the Big League and I wasn't sure if I was up to being a player. Because even though everyone who knew me thought I was super-confident, the truth is I wasn't.

On the surface, yes. I knew I wrote a column people connected with and liked. I knew I was a good interviewer and could make people tell me stuff they didn't even tell their family but it was a superficial confidence, the kind that could be knocked by even the smallest slight. I'm the kind of person, who if forty-eight out of fifty people said I was fantastic at my job I wouldn't listen – I'd be fretting about the two people who thought I was dreadful. And I don't think I'm alone in that. We're all driven, motivated by what other people think of us, there are very few people confident enough to ignore negative criticism.

Anyway, despite my fears I accepted the job. What kind of journalist would I have been to have said no to the chance of working for the world's biggest-selling newspaper? Besides the salary was HUGE – double the one I'd been earning at the *Sunday Mirror*. But it was with that salary that the pressure started to mount.

In my head and in my heart I didn't believe I was worth that kind of cash. What on earth could I possibly do to justify it? What would I have to produce, to achieve, to have my bosses think I was worthy of it? I was just a working-class Geordie girl from a Newcastle mining village. People like me didn't earn money like that, let alone deserve it. I spent my whole career thinking one day I'd be sussed. That people would realise I'd been winging it all these years.

I know now that was the start of the anxiety. It was always in the back of my head. Every word I penned, every column I wrote, every feature I produced, I would always ask myself: am I really worth what they're paying me? And the answer was always a resounding no.

Don't get me wrong, no-one would have thought for one minute that's how I was feeling. Not for a second. On the outside I was big, brash Carole. I never showed weakness, I never wanted anyone to know the insecure Carole that lurked inside – the one that was plagued with feelings of worthlessness. Don't get me wrong, if my boss gave me a rollicking for not doing something well, I didn't crumple. Because invariably he was right. I can always take criticism if it's something I deserve. And usually he didn't have to tell me a piece I'd written wasn't 100 per cent – I already knew, but had been hoping he might not notice. Colin Myler always did. But under him and on that newspaper I blossomed. I loved the fact the paper had clout, it had money. We always got the best stories, we were always on the side of the underdog.

It was a stellar time in my career. I believed and

had been told I would be there for the rest of my career, if I wanted to be. The security of that, for me, was fantastic. Over the years my friends had grown weary of me predicting that whatever newspaper I was working on at the time would fire me. Because I always believed I would be fired, that people would find me out. But at the *NOTW*, I felt safe.

That was until that sunny afternoon on 7 July 2011. I was at home in the garden when I got a phone call from a friend of mine at ITN, who told me the *NOTW* had just announced it was closing because of the phone hacking scandal. I couldn't believe it. A newspaper that had been running for 168 years – closed? How could that be? I couldn't take it in. My brain just wouldn't compute it. But in that instant my whole world fell in on me. The newspaper I loved was closing and with that was going my safety, my security and the security of 200 other journalists.

I immediately got in my car – I felt a compulsion to drive into the newspaper's offices in London to be with all my colleagues who'd just received this devastating news. But even as I was driving, listening to the news on the car radio, it still didn't feel real. It was like I was in a trance. My husband Nino was sitting alongside me and he kept asking why I was so calm (it's not a trait people usually associate with me!). And from the outside it probably looked like I was. But nothing could have been further from the truth. I was stunned. There was a part of me still refusing to believe what had just happened.

Once inside the newsroom I knew it was real. I could smell the panic, the fear. Stunned people were walking round with a combination of terror and disbelief etched onto their faces. People were literally shaking with fear. These people had families, mortgages, commitments, debts. You could see them all thinking, 'What the hell are we going to do?' All the people in that room had had nothing to do with the hacking, much of which had happened years before, but still, there we were, paying the price with our jobs.

So we did what all journalists do in times of trouble – we decamped en masse to the pub. And as I looked round, sipping my glass of house white (which tasted like vinegar, I was feeling physically sick), I remember wondering what would become of us all. In the space of a one short hour my career had gone from being as successful as it ever had been to dead in the water.

In the aftermath of the closure no one wanted to touch the *NOTW* journalists even though they knew we weren't involved in the scandal. I'd have to wait until everything had settled down. So in my mind a career of thirty-five years with some incredible highs was now down the toilet. At fifty-six years old I was finished. Untouchable. Unemployable.

I started to drink more than I should. And I ate more than I should – all the wrong things, obviously. I'd sleep for hours at a time for the simple reason I didn't want to be awake and face the horrible reality of my life. People told me that, of course, I'd work again. That I was too talented not to. But in those early days the phone didn't ring. There were no offers of work. So I just ate and slept and felt sorry for myself.

Then I started to look at my friends who were working. And I was angry. I was angry that they had a job and I didn't. I was resentful. So I picked arguments with them. I thought if I fought with them enough they would all abandon me, which would make it easier to sink into the abyss into which I wanted to hide.

I used to say to my husband, who I'd pushed and pushed until he too was almost at the end of his tether, that the world would be better off without me. What was the point of me if I couldn't work?

I know people say 'Work is what you do, it's not who you are'. But for me it always had been who I am. I didn't who I was supposed to be if I wasn't Carole Malone the columnist, the commentator, the person on TV who was always shouting the odds about something. But all the time this was happening, all the time my self-esteem was plummeting off a cliff, something else was happening inside my body that just wouldn't allow me to function on any level. It wasn't just that I was piling on weight, I was terrifyingly irrational, unreasonable, hopeless and pretty much helpless too. I literally couldn't drag my body out of bed in the morning – not that I wanted to. And I was eating erratically, none of it good. I ate rubbish to fill the void. I did zero exercise (what was the point? I had nothing and I was going nowhere). Every morning I woke up in a fug of anxiety and panic. And every night I woke at some ungodly hour, obsessing about a future that looked empty and bleak.

And then one day a very dear friend suggested I might be suffering from depression. I all but bit her head off. How could she say that? I wasn't one of those 'weak' people who wallowed in self-pity, I didn't 'do' depression. So she left and when she'd gone, I realised that yes, I absolutely WAS one of those people. Something had taken hold of my body that I just couldn't control. And I was scared because I had no idea how to stop it.

When I talked to my husband he said I should see a doctor. I refused point-blank – I didn't need a doctor. But three weeks later, I was sitting in front of one, who explained to me what the imbalance of hormones, bad diet and too much alcohol can do. He told me low self-esteem can trigger depression but so too can fat and sugary foods, an excess of which can cause chemical changes in the brain because chemicals changed by diet are those associated with depression. This made total sense to me. For months I had been comfort eating, which for me meant cakes, chocolate, doughnuts and jelly babies. Anything that was bad for me, I shoved down my throat by the bucket load. I was being spiteful to myself – and I knew it. But I did it anyway.

Every day I got on the scales to find my weight creeping higher. But I didn't care. Racing down the road to self-destruction, I felt worthless: I had no job, no future, I'd alienated everyone who'd been close to me. Who cared if I was the size of a house? No one was looking at me anymore, that's for sure. When I did get offered TV jobs I turned them down. How could I go on-screen looking like this great big bloated failure? Which of course made me even more depressed, which in turn made me eat more.

The doctor had told me I should try a course of antidepressants. When I asked how long I'd need to be on them he said they could take a couple of months to kick in. And then I'd probably need to take them for six months or more after that. I remember listening to him and knowing without a shadow of a doubt that I was never going to take them. He'd told me this was the best way to regulate the chemicals in my brain and I have no doubt that this approach works successfully for vast numbers of people and that it's absolutely the right thing to do for them. But I knew that route wasn't for me – I didn't want to be taking drugs for a year of my life.

I decided that if I'd caused this depression by eating junk and drinking too much then I'd stop doing it and get back to the gym. And so I did. I changed my diet, I knocked the wine on the head and I went back to the gym. I won't say for a second it was easy. There were days when I thought I might have to run to the drawer where I kept the box of antidepressants the doctor had given me in case I decided I needed them. But in the end I always stopped myself. Because even though what I was doing was cripplingly hard, even though every day was like crawling out of a deep black hole half an inch at a time, I knew I didn't want to take the drugs. But slowly, and I mean slowly, I started to feel better.

It was incredible to me that just by changing my diet – eating protein, vegetables including dark leafy greens, fruit, nuts and low-fat dairy – the gloom began to lift. The feelings of worthlessness began to feel less severe. The spectre of hope raised its shiny head. I began to feel I might actually have a future after all; that I might be able to work again. Yes, there were days when I felt I might fall back into the black hole but then I'd go to the gym and that gave me the strength to go into the next day.

The point of telling you all this is that so much of what we are, so much of how we feel, is down to what we eat. And it's not just that you feel a sense of achievement when you've lost weight and are eating well. Physically, you feel entirely different: you feel energised, the aches and pains we all have recede. You feel a sense of wellbeing that makes you almost giddy. Your ability to cope with stressful situations is enhanced. Your thinking is clearer. You're less angry and more able to deal with life. The world looks and feels like a good place to be. And let's face it, who wouldn't want all that?

At various points in my life I've let everyone down with my weight. When I was fifteen and already a bit chunky my parents coughed up for me to join Weight Watchers. It doesn't sound like much but it was a big sacrifice for them. Back then we didn't have much money and cooking special Weight Watchers recipes just for me took a hefty portion of the weekly household budget.

I lost two stones with Weight Watchers (which was all I needed to lose) before I started cheating. And then one day my mum was cleaning my bedroom and I'd forgotten about the stash of Mars Bars papers hidden under my bed. She went bonkers – not least because they'd invested time and money in helping me. But the lure of a Mars Bar (well, quite a few Mars Bars, actually) proved to be too strong. And my parents were furious.

When I left home at nineteen and got a flat of my own I went to Slimming World. And that worked too – until I started to cheat. I then tried the Cabbage Soup Diet and the Grapefruit Diet. I even went on a Mars Bar diet, which involved eating three of them a day and not much else, but I even managed to cheat on that one as well and introduced cakes into the mix, which was a definite no-no. Then about twelve years ago I was chosen to do an ITV show called *Celebrity Fit Club*. I jumped at the chance because not only would I be getting paid, I knew that with the entire country watching me I couldn't cheat. And finally, finally, I would lose weight.

My fellow slimmers that year were Russell Grant, Anne Diamond and ITV's Sharon Marshall. There was also the lovely footballer Mickey Quinn (former Newcastle United player) and former World Champion darts player Bobby George. We all threw ourselves into the task. Every weekend we'd travel to a stately home outside London that ITV had hired and we'd be given lectures. Harvey Walden, the American Marine fitness trainer, would fly to London every Friday to put us through our paces at weekends. The regime was gruelling, especially so for me as I'd never done any proper exercise. It was Harvey who first introduced me to the gym. Yes, I'd taken out gym memberships in the past but I'd never actually used them – I went to the spa and the bar and not much else. But Harvey made it clear: either I got stuck in or I was off the programme. And anyone who remembers Harvey would know he doesn't mess about: you did what he told you or you were out. But not without a lot of pain and humiliation first.

And so for three months the nation would tune in and watch our progress. And mine was impressive: I lost three and a half stones. More importantly, I surprised even myself and became a gym bunny. Because we had just three months to lose weight we had to run at it. Every day I went to the gym and after the first few painful sessions I loved it. Well, actually that's not true: I loved what it did for me and how it made me look and feel.

I loved the fact if I burned 1,000 calories a day on the machines – and I did – I could eat whatever I liked and still be a size 12. But I also loved the fact I had conquered my fear of the gym. Because I realised that I had been frightened of it. One of the main reasons I'd never been a regular at the various gyms I'd joined was because I felt stupid, out of place. I felt like a great big heifer while everyone else around me was toned and fit. I thought they would laugh at me.

When I told Harvey this he just roared with laughter and said: 'This might be hard for you to understand, Carole, but no one's looking at you. No one's interested, they're all too busy working out.' But I knew that wasn't true because when I saw grossly overweight people trying – and very often failing – to get to grips with exercise in the gym, I looked. I looked at them and pitied them. And I knew they would look at me and feel the same. But after three months at the gym I was a different person. A bunch of incredibly beautiful and buff gay guys had taken me under their wing (they admitted they'd felt sorry for me when I first started) and they helped me shape and define my shrinking body. It wasn't just enough to burn calories, they told me, it was about getting definition. So I worked hard and yes, I got my definition. And I never looked so good.

It's hard to explain the sheer joy of walking into a shop after years of having to go to outsize outlets and buying anything with an elasticated waist and then being able to try on – and look great in – almost anything. In fact it was so joyous, so seductive, that I developed a bit of a shopping habit (addiction, more like!) that I've never quite managed to shake off. Because for the first time ever I was able to buy clothes that I loved, not just clothes that would fit me.

More importantly, I felt different. And because of that people treated me differently. I looked younger, I had energy, I wasn't angry with the world (fat people tend to be although they're really angry at themselves) and finally, I knew I was attractive – I saw people's response to me every day. And while I know looks and being a size 12 aren't all that's important in life, to someone who hadn't had either, it felt wonderful. You see, I'd had years of people telling me I had a lovely face and although I was grateful for that it was what they weren't saying that registered with me: great face, shame about the body.

People who've never been overweight can't know what it's like to go through life knowing you're nothing like the person you feel you should be; that you're not functioning as the man/woman that inside you know you truly are. And that the person the world sees when it looks at you isn't actually how you see yourself.

One way to describe it is that you go through life on half-throttle. It's like the battery's charged but something's stopping you from going as fast as you know you can. Something is stalling, dragging you back. You want to do a million things but the three, four five extra stone you're carrying won't let you.

I spent years saying to myself, 'I'll do that when I'm thin.' So, I got thin – well, thinnish. I started Fit Club at nearly sixteen stone and got down to thirteen in the three months it was on air. And so energised, so motivated was I by the whole experience that I carried on when it was over. I still went to the gym every day, I still ate healthily. In fact, I had no choice because every time I went to a supermarket people who'd watched the show were always looking in my trolley to see what I was buying. But it was good, it kept me on my toes and I felt they cared enough to will me on. So, two months later, I'd lost another two stone. For the first time in my adult life I was into size 12 jeans.

I wasn't skinny, I didn't look gaunt, I was just right – and I'd never felt healthier.

I remember thinking back then how stupid I'd been to have stayed so fat for so many years. How much time had I wasted feeling bad about myself? Feeling less of a person in the company of people who I thought were better than me simply because they were the right weight. How much of my life did I put off living because I was too scared/too embarrassed/too ashamed of my size? And so the next few years were fantastic. But of course you know what's coming: I self-sabotaged. It didn't just happen suddenly, it happened over the period of a year. I started going to the gym a bit less – three times a week instead of five. Then work got busy. I got that job at *News of the World* and life was hectic – too hectic to go to the gym five times a week. (You see the excuses we fatties make to ourselves for not doing what we know we should!)

The job – I was a columnist and interviewer – involved lots of travelling and entertaining. Lots of celebrity parties. Lots of champagne. And I threw myself into it all. Until one day it dawned on me that I wasn't going to the gym any day of the week and my jeans were tighter. My boobs were bigger too, much bigger. Even my shoes felt a bit tight (and yes, you can put weight on your feet).

So I got on the scales. I was a stone and a half heavier:

twelve and a half stone. But I didn't panic. 'I can get that off in six weeks,' I thought to myself. 'It's not a disaster.' I reminded myself that I'd lost five stone in total so it wasn't a train wreck. And I still looked thin. I was a size 14 – well, maybe 16 by then – but it was all very retrievable. But of course I didn't retrieve it, I just kept on eating and eating. Not in great big binges, but carelessly. More doughnuts than vegetables, more chocolate than pulses... More wine than sparkling water. And it wasn't long before I tipped the scales at thirteen stone four pounds.

I did panic then – I knew that if I shot back up to 16 stone then I'd be fat for the rest of my life. Losing weight would just seem like too big a mountain to climb. So I joined Lighter Life. OK, it's not a diet I'd recommend for the long term but in short term – for me, anyway – it worked wonders. I lost three and a half stone in three months. No, it wasn't always pleasant and I couldn't go to the gym as I didn't have enough energy. However, I know me and I knew I couldn't take a year to lose this weight. I had to hit the ground running and get it off fast otherwise my weak will would crack. And so that's what I did.

The truth is once you get used to not eating anything other than the bars and drinks and packets of food Lighter Life provides you get used to it. More importantly, the weight loss is so rapid and your shape changes so quickly that it gives you a massive incentive to stick at it. I lost ten pounds in my first week, seven in my second. So in just two weeks I looked entirely different. This time I got down to a size 10. Truth be told I was too thin. There has not been a time before or since that I've been able to say that, but this time I was TOO thin. I was ten stone four pounds and I realised my ideal weight was about eleven to eleven stone four.

Men told me I didn't look sexy as I was too skinny (they want curves apparently, the very curves I'd spent a lifetime trying to get rid of). Women – well, women reacted in two ways. There were those women who had always felt reassured by me being fat: I wasn't a threat, you see. Yes, my face was half-decent but I wasn't the full drop-dead package and they liked that – they liked the fact that I'd never be a real looker because of my body. Those women would sidle up to me at parties when I was in my over-the-knee black suede boots and my Dolce & Gabbana mini kilt and say in a concerned whisper, 'Are you alright?' Then there were my real friends, the ones who said, 'You've lost too much, you don't look like you.'

In the beginning I ignored them all. I was into size 10 J Brand jeans and they could all sod off! I was going to live that life for a while, the one where you throw on those jeans and a tight white T-shirt and you're good to go anywhere. And I went everywhere with that body. I had my own TV shows, I appeared regularly on other people's shows. My writing career was good, my marriage was good... life was good.

Everywhere I went people were telling me how fabulous I looked. I could wear bikinis on the beach and not feel ashamed. And even though I was – and still am – happily married, I got chatted up all the time, which, at my age, is pretty damn flattering. People who hadn't seen me for a long time would gasp and spend the next twenty minutes rhapsodising about how fabulous I looked. Of course I loved every minute of it. I'd waited my whole life to hear this stuff. SO WHY DID I GO AND COCK IT ALL UP? And why, after forty years of dieting, do I continue to do so?

★★★

The month I hit the big Six-Ø, my right hip started to hurt. The same month, I developed something called diverticulitis. The dull ache in my chest that had been there for months suddenly exploded into what I know is acid reflux. Oh, and did I mention that I'd let the weight creep back on soI was three and a half stones overweight and every flight of stairs felt like I was scaling the north face of the Eiger? And without being too dramatic about it I found myself constantly asking the question, 'Is this it?' I didn't have a full-blown depression but this wasn't me. I had this overwhelming feeling there had to be more to life. I had no energy, no oomph; the spark had gone. And for years, I'd relied on my spark: it helped propel me through the 35-year bare-knuckle ride that has been my journalistic career.

All this stuff was swirling around in my head in the first three weeks of October. In the fourth week my consultant told me I'd have to have my right hip replaced. I was furious. Affronted. People my age don't get their hips replaced, they don't get weird ailments called diverticulitis. In fact, I actually told the consultant who delivered this irritating diagnosis that she'd made a mistake. *I don't get things like that,* I told her. All this stuff happens to other people, *old* people. And then it hit me. I was – officially, at least – a pensioner. That thing I thought would never happen to me (in my twenties I thought every sixty-year-old should be taken to a clinic far, far away and euthanised). I never expected to get old, to feel it – worse still, to look it.

For years people have told me I don't look my age. The really kind ones have said I look ten years younger. And in my head I believed I was. I scrubbed up well so when I needed to look good, I did. But most of the time I looked a mess and was trying to cope with the realisation that all the things I thought weren't going to happen to me for another ten years WERE happening. And all at once.

It was a hammer blow to my vanity, my confidence, my sense of self. I'd spent thirty-odd years as a journalist, which required spark and self-confidence. It required me to feel good about myself so that I was able to get what I needed to get from others. And for a long time it all worked beautifully. I got married at thirty-seven to an incredible man, who loved me whether I was fat or thin. My career was now going from strength to strength, both in newspapers and on TV. For some bizarre reason and despite the years of yo-yo dieting, my face rarely put on weight so for much of the time I was able to hide exactly how fat I was. But – and I've never actually said this out loud because it would sound vain – I had a big personality. So whatever I lost in the body stakes I made up for with the personality. And best of all, barring a bit of a bad back, I was healthy. And for thirty-five years all that worked for me even though I always took the 'spark', the personality, for granted and used it to great effect in my job.

And even if I did get way too fat – The Husband pointed out one day that I was the same weight as the England rugby prop forward we were watching on telly – someone would offer me a TV show which challenged me to lose three stones in three months, which I always did. Because to me that was a job and although I never put much effort into my body, I always put effort into my work.

I travelled the world, I was forever jumping on planes. I had boundless energy. I loved what I did. But then at sixty, I ran head-on into the wall and everything changed, literally overnight.

I know now it wasn't my actual age. There are lots of fabulously healthy sixty-year-olds walking around who DO look years younger. But in my case it was my body sounding the alarm after years of abuse, of taking my good health for granted. Of eating rubbish, of not doing enough exercise. For the first time ever I actually felt my age. I felt heavy not in terms of poundage (although that was the case), but it was like I was carrying some huge weight on my shoulders. I was anxious all the time – even in my sleep. I woke up anxious. I'm a short-tempered person but my mood swings were now out of control. Anything could make me lose it – stupid things like someone taking a parking space, someone looking at me the wrong way (in my head I thought they were judging me and looking down on me). No one outside knew, not even my friends, how I was feeling – I always managed to pull the 'full-of-fun Carole' out of the bag when we were out. But inside I knew I was losing it.

I thought everything would get better if I lost some weight. And I DID try, but it just wouldn't budge and even when I did lose a few pounds (on a starvation diet with a bit of gym thrown in), I'd put it straight back on when I came off the diet. But worse than being fat was the way I felt. The spark had gone from my eyes and from my very being. That lust for life which for years had propelled me through it at one hundred miles an hour was also gone. I felt dead inside. And fat. And ugly. And the crazy thing was, I didn't much care. I didn't have the energy to care. But I DID have the energy to worry about stupid, unimportant stuff.

Added to everything that was going on in my head and inside my body my mobility was severely limited because of the hip. I'd had an MRI scan, which as well as telling me that my hip was badly affected with arthritis (who knew I had that, for God's sake?), it also said I had a touch of it in two of my discs. I'd been aware of a bit of back pain and the fact a couple of my fingers were a bit achy, but I never ever gave it any thought because it wasn't that bad and I thought that's just what happens when you get older – aches and pains. But it was there. And I know now it was another indicator, another way of my body telling me I had to change what I put into it. But much more importantly, I know now it can be cured (more about that later).

Back to the hip... As I was limping around London I noticed that people walking past me refused to help me or give me space (I guess it was because I looked and was behaving like someone who was old). I felt like wallpaper – there but with no one really noticing me. Also, I had the constant, nagging urge to cry. The Carole Malone of just two years ago would never have allowed people to push past her in the street, to dismiss her, to treat her with such disrespect. But it was happening. And one day I looked in the mirror and I knew why.

I looked beaten because of the constant pain in my hip (and the knees and the back). But worse my eyes looked dead, which was about right because I felt dead inside. I wasn't fat, glamorous and funny anymore, I was just fat. And it made me look old. I had a great big spare tyre round my middle. I walked with a limp. The face that had always saved me looked tired. If I caught my reflection in a window it was one of someone I didn't recognise. I felt like I was operating on 50 per cent of what I was capable of, but I had no idea how to restore the 50 per cent of me that I'd lost.

And then I met Dr Aamer Khan. I'd gone to him thinking he could give me some Botox, fillers to rejuvenate my tired old face. We talked and I told him how I was feeling and then he suggested I have some tests. Specifically, DNA tests and adrenal stress tests (through saliva) and parasitology (stool) tests. He referred me to a nutritionist – Angela Beechcroft – who talked to me about what I ate, my lifestyle, and my feelings. And so I had the tests and the results were mind-blowing. Angela told me that in fifteen years she hadn't seen cortisol levels as high as mine, which were THREE TIMES the normal limit. So she gave me an eating programme to follow, which she said would take away the inflammation in my body.

So I ate everything I knew I was going to have to give up – pizza, cream cakes, chocolate, almond croissants and jelly babies. I had the lot! Then I went to bed on Sunday night fit to burst (we've all done it) in anticipation of the torture that was to come. But because I felt so stuffed and greedy and revolting I was also ready to start to change my life. Wasn't this feeling of being fat and bloated what I hated? Isn't that what sapped my self-confidence, made me feel like a big ugly blob?

How could I do that? Good question. But it's what I've been doing for years: I get to a good body weight, I'm happy, I feel good. I've bought lots of (small) beautiful clothes. People tell how fantastic I'm looking. Then something happens in my life and BOOM! I'm head-first into a bucket of carbohydrates. BOOM again and I'm diving into a bucket of sugar. It's been the cycle that's plagued my life. I don't want to be fat, I actually hate being fat, so why do I always end up that way? Why do I do this to myself – eat foods that I KNOW will make me pile on the stones? It's like I have a self-destruct button in my head which says, 'Yep, you think you've got it all going for you, girl. Well, take THIS!' And I'm a size 20 in elasticised pants before you can say Krispy Kreme doughnut.

I don't know why I do it – take refuge in the foods

I know are killing me. But I do know that in times of terrible stress, when life throws me a curveball, the cakes, the sweets and the bread are in some twisted terrible way a comfort to me. So why is that? Why is a doughnut so soothing when a nice crispy salad is not? Why does an apple crumble make me feel all warm and cosy inside when a baked apple does nothing for me?

All my life food has been my friend and my enemy simultaneously. If I've had a bad day there has been joy in knowing that when I get home there's a bakewell tart waiting for me. When I'm upset, I buy a box of chocolates to 'make me feel better'. But it doesn't. Because when I've finished them, I'm still upset. And I'm more depressed because now I'm feeling greedy and out of control as well.

And then my hip went and it was a wake-up call. It wasn't being fat that made the cartilage disappear but it WAS what made walking, moving about, getting out of a chair excruciating painful and difficult. I knew then things had to change but I didn't know how. I seemed to be constantly on a diet but never losing weight. I'd lose three pounds in a week – a change from twenty years ago when I could shed half a stone in seven days – and then have one night out and it was all back on again.

I'd been on so many diets I thought I knew how to do it – clearly, I didn't. But then I met Dr Aamer and his wife Lesley and as I've said they suggested I have some tests that would determine what was going on with my body. They referred me to nutritionist Angela Beechcroft, who organised Adrenal Stress profile tests and stool tests. And the results were astounding.

The reason I hadn't been able to lose weight became clear. Angela said it was because my cortisol levels were THREE times as high as they should be. In her fifteen years as a nutritionist she had rarely seen levels as high as mine. Which was actually terrifying because cortisol is what's often called the 'stress hormone' (it influences, regulates and modulates many of the changes that occur in the body's responses to stress). High levels can cause heart attacks, strokes, diabetes, high blood pressure and osteoporosis. It can also cause anxiety and mood swings, two conditions that have plagued me for years. What has also plagued me for the past five years is a great big fat tyre around my middle which refuses to budge. Angela told me my sky-high cortisol was responsible for this too – mine and the spare tyres of millions of other women. And it's this abdominal fat which is particularly dangerous as it can cause heart attacks and strokes. It is also high levels of cortisol that hang onto this fat and, as Angela told me, 'With levels this high, you will never lose an ounce.' Talk about a wake-up call!

Faced with that, I had no choice: life had to change – and fast. Because at sixty how many more years could I put it off? I'm lucky that so far (and I'm touching wood here) life, in terms of my health, has been kind. But the results of those tests made me realise there could be no more 'I'll start on Monday' weeks. Because this wasn't just about dieting or losing weight, this was no longer just dropping a couple of dress sizes, but literally saving my life. It was about turning back time, stopping the ageing clock; knowing that taking control could make me twenty years younger inside. I could stop the heart attack which, according to my genetic code, is lying in wait. I could prevent the stroke, the osteoporosis, the anxiety that often grips my body like a vice...

So, breakfast on Day One, I wasn't in the least bit hungry – truth be told, I was still stuffed from the night before. But I knew I had to have the breakfast smoothie as it was the only way my system was going to be cleansed. That said, it wasn't a happy affair. I had the decorators in, so the breakfast smoothie was made on top of dustsheets and trying to gather the ingredients which had all been moved out of my cupboard. I'd like to say the smoothie – blueberries, flaxseed, cinnamon, ginger root, coconut milk – tasted great, but it didn't. It tasted like medicine. But I figured that's exactly what it was. So I took my medicine. It wasn't the same as a bowl of Special K or a buttered bagel, but as I've learned throughout the years, feeling good, fit and a normal dress size doesn't come without hard slog. And this time around, I wasn't even off the starting block.

Lunch (boiled eggs and salad and homemade soup) and dinner (fish and salad) was all fine. I went to bed feeling virtuous. The next morning I got weighed and had lost TWO pounds! Which is one way to make the medicinal smoothies go down a bit better.

The next few days I was hungry – I was eating all my meals AND my mid-morning and mid-afternoon protein snacks, but I felt like my body was actually burning fat for the first time in as long as I can remember.

The first week my energy levels were low. Angela had warned that I could feel worse before I got better – she was right. Walking up stairs was hard. I had no energy, pain everywhere.

When I got to Week Six I had been doing really well. Then I realised that the following weekend Nino and I would be attending a ball in Dorset. The upside was that I'd lost ten pounds and I was a dress size smaller so the usual 'I've Got Nothing To Wear' panic on the night would be a bit less frantic. First, because the midriff bulge that had stuck steadfastly with me for the past year was ever so slightly smaller. And second, because having broken two toes a month before (that's a whole other story!), I couldn't wear my heels and so I had the perfect excuse to wear baggy evening trousers and black sparkly FitFlops.

So at least the outfit was sorted. The terrifying thing was that I knew this was going to be a boozy night – champagne reception, three course dinner. How on earth was I going to stick to the plan? Dr Aamer always says not to panic about these occasions, just be as good as you can be. What he couldn't have bargained for was Malone's infamous and shameful lack of willpower. And the fact that all good sense and intentions go flying out the window when you're onto your third toffee vodka shot!

You see I'd never had toffee vodka before or any kind of flavoured vodka for that matter. It just tasted sweet and lovely and innocuous. I'd started the night well at a friend's with a couple of glasses of champers. Then I had a couple more at the reception. But the real trouble started when we sat down for dinner in this amazing marquee. There were fairy lights everywhere, and I was ever so slightly tipsy. The first course came – roasted tomatoes and bruschetta. At that point I still had enough sense to realise that the bread was a no-no, so I just ate the tomatoes. I ticked the 'Good Girl' box in my head on that. Then I had a couple of glasses of (forbidden) wine – it was awful, but I persevered. Next came the main course – bland chicken breast on a bed of veg. Everything might have been different had I eaten that. But at that point I was engrossed in conversation with a very handsome man who sells expensive cars so I forgot to eat anything and I just kept on drinking. And then came the toffee vodkas. I vaguely remember hearing my best friend tell me to step away from the vodka. I heard her telling me I didn't normally drink hard spirits so why would I start now when I was on this programme? Suffice to say I didn't listen and I drank hers as well when she popped to the loo.

But in the end it was a fantastic evening (I even cracked open a bottle of Prosecco with an amazing Canadian businesswoman who at that point I was determined was going to be my best friend for life). The next day was uglier than I could ever have believed possible. Never in my whole life had alcohol affected me the way it had that night. Don't get me wrong, I have had hangovers. I have drunk too much and felt a bit iffy the next day. But never, never did I throw up and feel as bad as I did that day. I threw up in the night; I threw up three times before I was able to go downstairs for breakfast. Then again when I had to leave the breakfast table. And then twice on the way home when The Husband had to stop so I could stick my head in a bush and throw up some more. I kept thinking as I heaved into what was a magnificent blackberry bush that here I was at sixty-one looking like some old lush. All the while I was trying to work out why I was so ill. Because although I'd drunk a fair bit of alcohol, I'd done it before. But never had it had this kind of effect on me. Never had the sickness been so virulent. And I realised that before that night my system had been pretty much clean. I'd had six weeks of eating only the best and the purest of foods. I'd had only the tiniest amount of alcohol. I'd been piling probiotics into my body to improve the bacteria in my gut. I'd purged myself of all the crap and in one night I'd literally poisoned my nice clean body. And that body was telling me loud and clear that not only didn't it want this poison, it could no longer cope with it.

If there's an upside to this story it's that I didn't touch a drop of alcohol for the next three weeks. Just the mention of the word 'wine' conjured up visions of nasty vinegary things and me with my head in a bush throwing up. The other upside is that of course I lost a pound that weekend, but I know that's not the way to do it.

This was one of the many lessons I learned on this programme. I wasn't just working hard to lose weight this time, I was working hard to try and get my insides functioning the best possible way they could. And in one crazy (wonderful!) night I'd wrecked that. It took two whole days of vegetable smoothies and omelettes and light food to make me feel well again.

WEEK NINE

I'm stuck. I've lost 16 pounds and it's like God has decreed that's my lot. I've been this weight for three weeks now. For one day only I slipped down to 13st 11lb (haven't been there for three years!), but then I went back up to 13st 12lb. And that's where I've stayed. The thing is, I've got into a way of eating that's OK but I'm getting bored now because I find myself eating the same stuff every day. I'm not changing anything, I'm not putting any variety into it, which is a mistake because in the past when I've gotten bored I dive headlong into a pan of chips. Yes, I've found some meals, some foods that I like, and I've stuck with them. And I'm not entirely sure that everything I'm doing is right.

Note to self: I need to see more of Dr Khan.

At the start I was convinced that I understood what I was doing. I had a couple of chats with the nutritionist and one with Dr Khan and then I thought, *I don't need any more help, I can do this on my own now.'* But the thing is, I'm trying to change a lifetime of catastrophically bad habits and I've realised I can't do it without step-by-step guidance. I'm aware that I've started including some foods that wouldn't necessarily be bad on any other diet, but on this one – they're forbidden. Stuff like Parma ham, semi-skimmed milk.

Dr Aamer came to our house this week to have a nose around my food cupboards because I think he thinks I'm doing something wrong. And his worst suspicions were confirmed. You see, I thought when they said I could eat rye bread that meant ALL rye bread. So I found this amazing soft, pillowy one at M&S that tastes divine (like liquid treacle). Dr Khan took one look at it and said, 'You can't have this.'

'It's rye bread,' I protested. And then he looked at the list of ingredients and pointed out the big fat word that said WHEAT. Now that's not fair. How can food manufacturers tell you you're buying rye bread and it's stuffed to the ginnels with wheat, which I'm not supposed to have? What kind of cruel maniac does that to someone who's busting a gut to change her life?

Dr Khan carried on plundering my cupboards and the rice cakes were thrown out as were the oatcakes, which I was convinced I could have. He found the semi-skimmed milk, which is also a no-no. He found the Green & Black's dark chocolate with bits of salt in it. Now that got a big fat tick (you can have four little squares of dark chocolate a day). But then he found the orange Kit Kats. You see I thought a single finger a day at just 45 calories was OK, but as he pointed out, this isn't about calories, it's what's in the food. Apparently there was nothing nutritious in my Kit Kats so into the bin they went. It got worse when he discovered an unopened box of fudge lurking in the back of a cupboard but I managed to convince him it was for dinner guests who wanted a bit of something sweet with coffee. They actually were for that, but there was no guarantee of course that I wouldn't fall upon them one night when I was feeling desperate and scoff the lot.

But the thing I have to tell you about this programme is that the craving for sugar actually does go away. I'm a sugar junkie. My whole life has been about getting as much of the stuff down my throat as is humanly possible in as many delicious forms as I can find – cakes, biscuits, chocolate bars, fizzy drinks, desserts, doughnuts (*especially* doughnuts). Sugar was my comfort blanket. When I was happy, I needed a cake. And when I was sad, I desperately needed a cake – and some chocolate even more.

WEEK TEN – SATURDAY

CATASTROPHE! Didn't just fall off the wagon this week, I hurled myself off it at one hundred miles an hour. I ate spaghetti, pizza, chocolate... I drank wine. It was only one of each – apart from the wine. That was a glass every night. But there is a significance to this: I'm repeating age-old patterns. I know this is much more important than just a cheat or a blip or whatever people call it when they throw food into their mouths they absolutely know they shouldn't have. I know this is my old demons resurfacing, the little devils inside my head, who every time I get close to getting in control they pop out of the hell inside me to stop me. I get close to changing the way I look, the way I eat, I drop a few dress sizes and there they are, screaming, 'OH NO YOU DON'T, FAT GIRL! YOU WERE BORN TO BE FAT AND WE'RE GOING TO MAKE SURE YOU STAY THAT WAY.' The demons have been dormant these past few weeks. Yes, they've been nipping at me, annoying me, making me look at things I want to eat but know I can't. But I even managed to still their voices when I looked at cakes and chocolate because for the first time ever I was looking at that stuff and saying, 'No, I really don't want that.'

But here I am in Week Ten – a place I have been many times before but usually sooner than Week Ten – and the self-destruct button has been pushed. And for the life of me I don't understand why.

I was doing so well. Dr Aamer came to my house and told me I'd done brilliantly. And I know I look better. I've lost sixteen pounds and my bum has gone from being gargantuan to just Very Large. I can get on jeans and trousers that have been sitting redundant on hangers for the past three years. People are telling me how good I look, how my face looks thinner, how my skin is fresh and my eyes are sparkling. And what do I do? I go buy a HUGE pizza from M&S and have it with wine – three bloody glasses of it.

The next day you'd think I'd get up and say, 'Well, that was yesterday. Today is a brand new day.' But I don't. I watch The Husband preparing his kale and spinach smoothie and instead of telling him to give me a glass of it so I can wash away all those nasty pizza toxins, I go to the freezer and pull out a red onion and chive bagel and have it slathered in cashew nut butter (there's still a bit of me that's trying to hang on in there).

And as it dawns on me that I have totally buggared it all up I tell The Husband that I'd like (white) spaghetti Al Olio for dinner that evening (my excuse was that it WAS Saturday night and I hadn't cheated for weeks and this was a one-off). Obviously he pointed out that I'd been cheating for two whole days but I'd already put on my invisible earphones so I could hear nothing and to stop him jabbing away at my conscience.

No sooner had he gone to the supermarket to get the spaghetti for that night's dinner than I suddenly remembered the packet of Haribo Jelly Babies skulking at the back of a drawer since I started all this. I'd always known they were there but I'd been feeling so virtuous that they were never even a temptation. Until now I haven't even thought about them, let alone wanted them. Today, their very existence is burning a hole in my brain and I know with every fibre of my being that before the day is done I'm going to grab a handful. The demons were dancing a jig in my head now. I could hear them saying, 'We've got her, we've got her!'

Who are these evil creatures who refuse to let me look the best and be the healthiest I can be? Why won't they let me be? Is there something in me that says I don't deserve to look fabulous, that people like me aren't ever destined to reach their full potential?

I've been doing this all my life – getting close to the weight I want to be and then messing up. Or actually getting there and languishing in the glow of all the compliments, promising myself I'll never go back there again. Then within six months, I'm back.

All that stuff I ate these past few days – the pizza, the cake (yes, there was also an apple turnover involved) and a huge plate of spaghetti. Oh, and there was the wine. I've been told I can't have wine – maybe only one day a week. But this week I've been having a glass a night. It doesn't sound like a lot, but it's six glasses in a week I'm not supposed to have. I'm also allowed to have four or five pieces of dark chocolate three or four days a week. I've been having SIX squares every night, which actually wasn't too bad. But then at lunchtime I've been adding a few squares in there too.

WHAT IS HAPPENING TO ME? WHY AM I DOING THIS?

In the midst of all this I did a TV pilot for a new current affairs show. Usually these things are a nightmare because I can't find anything to wear that (a) looks good and (b) fits. I thought this time would be better because I've lost sixteen pounds and some of my prettier shirts now fit. So off I go and once at the studio the producer tells me to wear a plum coloured silk shirt I've brought with me.

It slips on easily enough. I walk into the studio and all around me on the walls are two-foot-high photos of me that were taken in 2007 when I was on *Celebrity Big Brother*. Even if I say it myself, I looked good. But back then I was two and a half stone lighter.

I was doing the pilot with Katie Hopkins and a lovely former *Blue Peter* presenter Ayo Akinwolere. Katie, of course, is whippet-thin – fresh from putting on and then losing three stone just to prove that all it takes to lose weight is determination and willpower. More importantly, to prove that obesity is not a disease, it's something we wilfully do to ourselves.

So there we are, side by side: one woman who has the willpower of steel and another with the willpower of a gnat. She looks svelte and elegant, I'm a great big billowing bag of plum silk. Within a few minutes we are recording and I suddenly get a glimpse of myself on camera. God, I look HUGE. I'd forgotten that telly puts on at least ten pounds (funny how it doesn't on people who are already skinny) and so I looked as fat as ever. Depressing, depressing, depressing!

Just to compound the damage I went into a pub with The Husband at the weekend and told him to get me a bag of crisps. He looked at me much like a parent would look disapprovingly at a child who had just taken her knickers off in the street.

'Really?' he said. 'Really?' I hit back at him with the determination of a woman who is cutting off her nose to spite her face, determined to do her worst – to herself.

And do you know, those bloody crisps tasted awful. The first I've had in ten weeks (I used to have them every night with wine before dinner) and they tasted greasy and fatty and just... yuck! The glass of Whispering Angel rosé (the palest of pale roses) I had with it didn't taste in the least bit awful. Truth be told it was divine! But I think that's a cross I'm just going to have to bear. I love wine but I have to accept that for most of the week I just can't have it – the crisps, though, I now know I can happily give up.

Just a note about the pizza: I know when we cheat it feels like we are being driven to do so by a force greater than ourselves. And with me over the years it's been the guilt in my head that has stopped me doing it again. But now I know it's going to be something different that will stop me. Because after weeks of what I suppose I'd call 'clean' eating the pizza tasted fantastic at the time but the way I felt within half an hour of eating it wasn't quite so fantastic – I felt dirty and greasy inside, like the food was sticking to my gullet. I saw a blob of grease from the cheese had dropped on my jumper and as I watched the grease pool spread I thought, 'That's what's happening inside me.' I felt repulsed by myself and what I had done. Even my gullet felt sore and bruised by the doughy heaviness of it all. I also felt my acid reflux coming back.

I hadn't eaten dough in TEN weeks and although I had no problems eating it (at the time, it felt rather good), twenty minutes later I felt like it was sticking inside me. It just wouldn't digest properly. I went to bed bloated and feeling that old depression, that old hopelessness about my body return.

I'd lost control and I don't know how to get it back. And even as I'm writing this I'm not really sure that I'm back in control, that I won't cheat today or tonight. There are still some of those Jelly Babies left and I can't be sure that I won't think, 'What the hell?' and dive on them. The Husband's away this week so I don't have him to tell me off or to be my conscience.

What the hell is wrong with me?

★★★

17 November 2016. Not too bad a day today. Got out of bed at the crack of dawn (well, 6am) to get into town to meet Dr Khan at 7.30am. Boy, these healthy people start work early! He tells me not to feel too guilty about my

crazy few days: 'It happens,' he says. 'It's done, now get over it.'

Easier said than done, of course. This is a man who at university used to be an athlete with fitness in his very handsome genes. He takes off his jacket to reveal a svelte torso in a crisp white shirt. I remove my black sweater to reveal a T-shirt and exercise pants, which he told me to wear as Spencer Hayler (the personal trainer and coach) and I were going to have our first session.

I was not looking forward to that. Spencer is the byword for health and fitness. He lives and breathes health and it shows in his body. I don't like working out with perfect people – it makes me feel even more of a freak. However, I can't be the first fatso he's trained and I'm sure I won't be the last.

There's two big straps with handles hanging from the ceiling which he says we're going to use to do a circuit. And so we do. First, I do lunges with the aid of the straps. The cartilage in my right knee is split in two places from my stint on *Celebrity Fit Club* ten years ago when I collapsed on a running track after sprinting out of those starting blocks. Since then every couple of years the knee goes into meltdown for a couple of weeks and then it's OK-ish again.

I realise doing these exercise that my three months of Pilates has stood me in good stead. When I started I had no idea what my core was or where it was located. Now I understand what it is and how to use it and in these exercises Spencer was taking me through I needed to know what I was doing. But the straps were a huge help – they allowed me to do things I would not ordinarily have been able to do.

I did an exercise that involved something called planking; I did lunges and exercises to strengthen my back and arms. And actually, I loved it. That one session with Spencer had evaporated my fear of one-to-one sessions with handsome trainers – I was too busy concentrating on what I was doing to feel embarrassed.

OK, I know one exercise session isn't enough to change anything in my body but what it did do was to reboot my mind-set. I'd been flailing about for days, not knowing how to get back on track, and this exercise session did it. Because with every exercise I mastered, I began to see what was possible if I stuck to the plan. And there is absolutely no point in sweating and working out for an hour and then blowing it all with a doughnut and full-fat latte. So today was the day I got back on track. And it felt good. It's like my brain has been on a big seesaw, swishing about, not knowing what's happening. But now it's settling; it's getting back its equilibrium.

SEPTEMBER 2017

Well, I did it. I did what I always do: I self-sabotaged. At the start of the summer I'd lost fifteen pounds, I had energy, I had verve, all my aches and pains had virtually disappeared. OK, the big fat spare tyre that had steadfastly clung to my middle for the last few years hadn't entirely gone but it was smaller. Dr Aamer told me he was happy with my progress. He said I had a long way to go but at least I was on the way.

And that was great news, or at least it should have been. But I got cocky. I decided that as I'd been doing so well I could allow the odd chocolate in. A dessert now and then. A few carbs at lunchtime, which turned into two lovely bread buns every day bursting with salami and salad. Then I allowed myself the odd piece of cake. But it didn't matter because I kidded myself that I was still in control. And for the first few weeks I didn't put much weight on, even with the added treats. Yes, the weight loss stopped but I was maintaining, which was OK because I thought that gave me a free pass to cheat for a few weeks (this is how the mind of a fat person operates). But of course with all those added treats the maintaining suddenly turned into gaining.

And then it happened. That little trigger inside my head that says 'Sod It' kicked in. I made all the usual excuses; I told myself I'd start properly next week.

There were months to sort myself out before the book was due to be handed in.

I had a holiday coming up so I thought I'd wait until a few weeks before then – I'd go hell for leather so I'd be in good shape. I rationalised there was no way I'd let myself go to the beautiful hotel my husband Nino and I visit every year in Puglia, Italy, looking like a beached whale. But of course that's exactly what happened. Of the fifteen pounds I'd lost I put EIGHT back on. The spare tyre was back with a vengeance. And as well as feeling utterly miserable, I was also feeling sheepish and stupid.

Why on earth did I keep doing this to myself?

I didn't tell Dr Khan what was happening because I felt too ashamed. He and his wife Lesley had invested so much time and effort in me I felt I'd let them down. But this is my pattern: I recognise it, it's part of me.

It's not because I'm stupid, it's not because I'm uneducated about food. These days I know everything about it and I know what it takes to lose weight and keep it off. I'm not one of those people who doesn't know why I put weight on. I don't blame my genes, my parents, my childhood or Uncle Tom Cobley for the fact that I'm fat. I'm fat because I like cake and sweeties and pizza. And I know that to get or keep weight off either I stop eating that stuff or at least cut it down drastically.

And there have been many periods in my life where

I've done exactly that. But then I flick the Trigger Switch and take a springboard dive into the Carbs. There's obviously something in me that says I don't deserve to look good, that I don't deserve to reach my full potential. And so I spend my whole life feeling less of the person I think I should be. You see I have a vision in my head of the woman I think I was born to be. The Fantasy Me is a size 12 (and I was there for a while). She's in good shape, her muscles are taut, her arms devoid of bingo wings. She works out three times a week. She's happy, good natured and serene – she has the kind of serenity that comes from believing you're the best you can be.

The Real Me is a whole different story. I'm a size 18. My muscles scream if I have to walk up a slight incline. My arms DO have bingo wings. And I'm rarely serene. Just to give you an idea how far from serene I am Dr Aamer tested my serotonin levels and delivered the news that never in his career had he seen serotonin levels as high as mine. I'm supposed to wake up with a level of 28-something and I wake up with a level of 95. He told me I spend my life literally living on the edge, which negates the faintest chance of serenity. Or weight loss. Because stress and anxiety mean you hang onto your weight, especially the fat around your middle. Dr Aamer told me I had to get those levels down ASAP before any of my weight would come off.

The thing is – and those of you who, like me, have struggled for years with their weight will know this – if you look good and feel good, you put a certain face on to the world. And the world responds kindly to it. You walk along a street and people smile at you for no reason. You go into a store and the assistant wants to help. You buy a coffee and the barista instead of barely acknowledging you behaves like he/she's your friend. I'm not saying for a minute people respond in this way because you're thin, it's because there's an aura about you. Put simply, you're giving out good vibes because you're happy with yourself and people respond to that. But it doesn't mean you're walking around with a silly big grin on your face 24/7, what it means is you're at peace with yourself and people want to be around that. And I wanted to feel like that again ...

DECEMBER 2017

So here I am again. For the umpteenth time in my life I've lost weight and it's fantastic. I'm feeling better, looking younger. My clothes fit. I'm getting compliments again. I have energy, my joints don't hurt, the arthritis I've noticed in a couple of my fingers has gone. Best of all, the world feels like a nicer, kinder, happier place. Or maybe it's just my mind-set that's in a nicer, happier place.

But I've been here before and I'm not daft enough to think I won't ever mess up again. That I won't self-sabotage. That I won't just forget how good I feel now and dive into a bucket of Haribo jelly babies. Because for the last forty years I feel like I've been programmed to fail. Having said all of that, this time round there's a difference. This time it's about much more than my weight, how I look and what dress size I am: it's about what's going on inside me. My organ health. My blood health. My moods. My emotions. My anxiety. My energy levels. Also, I now know why my body seemed so determined to hang onto the spare tyre of fat around my middle for so long. It was because my cortisol levels were sky-high, thanks to work-related stress and anxiety.

Now, the truth is while in my profession a bit of anxiety, a bit of adrenaline is good for the performance, too much sends me racing to La La Land, with mood swings, hyperactivity and depressive feelings. It feels like I'm hurtling towards a cliff edge and I can't stop. That's how it's been with me these last few years and I hated it. I hated feeling out-of-control. It was a new and terrifying phenomenon for me. And one I didn't know how to cope with. Worse, I didn't know why it was happening.

In my twenties, thirties, forties and even my early fifties I used to positively thrive on stress, I loved the adrenaline rush of my job. But as I got older it became harder to cope with. In fact, I grew scared that I might not be able to cope with it. But Dr Khan helped me find out what was happening and he discovered the culprit was my cortisol levels, which trigger anxiety, mood swings and yes, weight gain. They were five times higher than they should be and so the eating programme and an assortment of supplements has corrected that.

So now I have my control back and I know that by eating certain things, taking certain supplements, I can stop those cortisol levels in their tracks. I also know that just by eating the right things I can take years not just off the body the world sees, but off the one it doesn't. I can literally Turn Back Time INSIDE. I can make my sixty-two-year-old body function like that of a forty-five-year-old. Now that's a much bigger, more important goal than getting three stone off for a holiday, or to fit into a new outfit for a friend's wedding.

This programme is about TURNINNG BACK TIME or, more accurately, it's about adding years to your life – GOOD years when your joints don't ache, when you can move easily. For me it's about not having to live with chronic acid reflux, with arthritis. It's about having my heart and brain function better than they might have before I changed the way I eat.

I've never bought the argument 'I'm fat because of my genes', I've always known I'm fat because I eat too many cakes, too much chocolate and too many carbs. But there was always a part of me that desperately wanted to believe it was my genes. That because my dad had been overweight and had, like me, battled all his life to control it, I had to have a genetic tendency towards obesity as well. But Dr Khan blew that theory out of the water. He said that 80 per cent of what we are is determined by environment and only 20 per cent is genetic. So now I know there can be no more excuses. That God didn't make me like this. My genes didn't, nor did the universe: I did it all by myself.

I wish I could tell you all now I will never be fat again. I wish I could say I have once and for all conquered my love of sweets and cakes and pizzas. But I can't. Because I'm human and humans make mistakes. They let themselves down. What I can tell you is that I would be one twenty-four-carat fool if I let myself spiral out of control again. Because now I have the elixir for a long and pain-free life. Now I know what I need to do – not just to stay a healthy weight but to feel well inside and out. Now I know that by eating the right things for my body I can lessen the chances of getting what my dad had and what his mum had – heart disease.

What kind of an idiot would I be if I ignored everything that, thanks to Dr Khan, I now know about my body – precisely what vitamins it needs and those it doesn't? Now I know what kind of foods my body craves and what kind it hates (sadly, they are the foods I love). I know the foods that will bring the weight and cause the inflammation and the joint pain to come crashing back.

What I need to keep track of are my 'Triggers' – those things that send me careering down the road of self-sabotage. For me I've learned those triggers can be set off by disappointments in my career, fears about money and security and insecurities within myself.

Turning sixty was a huge trigger for me because instead of thinking 'I really need to look after myself now,' my reaction was 'What's the point? The best part of my life is over, it's all downhill from here.' And as trite and as stupid as that sounds, it actually isn't. I know people keep saying 'Sixty is the new fifty' and that 'Age is just a number', but for a woman I think it's much more than that.

For me it felt like the end of something. Not my life, obviously. And while I'll be shouted down by The Sisterhood for not being more positive about the inevitability of ageing – the hellish and unavoidable truth is that it IS the end of something. It's the end of looking and seeing yourself as a sexual being. When I was young I liked the fact people looked when I walked into a room. I liked it when men found me attractive. And I don't care if that makes me sound vacuous and silly: it's a fact, it gave me confidence. That doesn't happen when you're sixty. Men and women don't look at me anymore and think 'Gorgeous', they think 'She's good for her age'. Your sexuality, your allure, is dimmed. You go from being a sixty-watt woman to a twenty-watt one. You become indistinguishable in a crowd. When a sixty-something woman tells people she's still working and has a good career there's often a surprised look on their faces that says, 'Why would you still be working now? You're done, aren't you, defunct?'

No one actually says it, but younger people DO think it. 'You must be ready to retire soon,' they say with sympathy in their eyes, like you're some pathetic creature who doesn't know when to let go.

So, yes, sixty is THE big milestone for many women because the horrible, indisputable truth is that when a woman hits that age her best years ARE behind her. And that didn't sit well with me. And I know it doesn't sit well with millions of other women who society mentally – and often physically – chucks on the scrap heap. So, and here comes the positivity bit, I was determined it wasn't going to be the end for me. OK, so George Clooney and Gerard Butler aren't ever going to be fighting over me. Gorgeous thirty-something men aren't going to be looking at me and thinking 'Hottie'. I can't flirt in the way I used to just in case people laugh at me. But I'm not going to not go for jobs because of how old I am. And the one thing I know for sure is that I'm very definitely not finished. For me it ain't over until the Fat Lady – or in my case, The Not So Fat Lady, sings. So now, after a lifetime of yo-yo dieting, my body's not bad. But it's my mind, my emotions, my mood, my general feeling of wellbeing that's exciting. Living a long life is going to be fabulous if I feel as good as this.

So to all of you embarking on this journey, this adventure, this lifesaving programme, I wish you love, luck and a long healthy life. It won't always be easy but stick with it. And even if you do fall off the wagon, clamber back on quick before the aches come back. Don't forget hunger isn't your worst enemy, it's your friend. If you don't feel it, you aren't losing weight.

And most of all remember what the great big glittering goal is: it means you can do what no other being – earthly or otherwise – can do.

I suppose what I'm saying is that you can make yourself the person you want to be just by eating the right things.

Try it...

You can Turn Back Time!

Carole Malone

December 2017

Acknowledgements

I would like to thank Carole for her collaboration, Jaine Brent my wonderful patient agent for helping me to fulfil my ambition of writing this book, to all the clients who have participated in this regime, to Despinda and Lucas for helping me to put the training and exercise programmes together and most of all my loving and patient wife Lesley who has kept me to the deadlines and her wonderful contribution to the recipes.

Dr Aamer Khan

I'd like to say a huge thank you to Lesley and Aamer for putting me on the right path. To my wonderful agent Jaine Brent who drove and supported me in equal measure. And to my husband Nino who has walked through this life with me through the 'thin' and the 'fat' times, putting up with the heady highs and hellish lows of both while always making sure I knew he loved me – whatever I weighed.

Carole Malone